THE ESSENTIALS OF HEALTH CARE OF THE ELDERLY

Gerald Bennett, MB, MRCP (UK)

Consultant in Health Care of the Elderly, The Royal London Hospital (Mile End), London

and

Shah Ebrahim, DM, MSc, MRCP (UK), MRCGP, MFCM, DCH

Professor and Honorary Consultant in Health Care of the Elderly,
The London Hospital Medical College and St Bartholomew's Hospital Medical College

Edward Arnold
A division of Hodder & Stoughton
LONDON   MELBOURNE   AUCKLAND

© 1992 Gerald Bennett, Shah Ebrahim

First published in Great Britain 1992

British Library Cataloguing in Publication Data
Bennett, Gerald C.J.
   The essentials of health care of the elderly.
   I. Title II. Ebrahim, Shah
   362.1

   ISBN 0–340–54559–3

Typeset in 10/11$\frac{1}{2}$pt Ehrhardt by Saxon Group, Derby.
Printed and bound in Great Britain for Edward Arnold, a division of Hodder and Stoughton Limited, Mill Road, Dunton Green, Sevenoaks, Kent TN13 2YA by Butler & Tanner Ltd, Frome and London

CONTENTS

FOREWORD   ix

PART ONE   ESSENTIALS OF AGEING

 1   Ageing: populations, organisms and cells   3

 2   Ageing skin   11

 3   The ageing eye   15

 4   The ageing ear   19

 5   The ageing kidney   22

 6   Ageing bone, muscles and joints   25

 7   The ageing brain   31

 8   The ageing cardiovascular system   35

 9   The ageing respiratory system   38

10   The ageing endocrine system   42

11   The ageing alimentary system   45

12   The ageing immune system   50

13   The ageing psyche   52

PART TWO   ESSENTIAL MEDICINE OF OLD AGE

14   The history of geriatric medicine   57

15 The elderly in society   61

16 Social networks   67

17 Presentation of disease   70

18 History-taking and examination: helping your elderly patient
    to help you   74

19 Immobility   83

20 Falls   87

21 Confusion   91

22 Incontinence   97

23 Pressure sores   103

24 Accidental hypothermia   108

25 Joint contractures   113

26 Depression   118

27 Psychotic and other disorders   124

28 Palliative care   128

29 Better prescribing   133

30 Elder abuse and inadequate care   137

31 Ethnic elders   141

32 Legal aspects   145

33 Stroke   150

PART THREE   SERVICES FOR ELDERLY PEOPLE

34 The multi-disciplinary team   157

35 Comprehensive health care   162

36 The day hospital   167

37 Severe chronic disability   170

38   Prevention in old age   176

39   Seeing patients at home   180

40   The elderly patient in Accident & Emergency   184

41   Discharge from hospital   188

42   The roles of team members   192

Index   209

FOREWORD

Prof Peter H. Millard M.D., F.R.C.P.,
Eleanor Peel Professor of Geriatric Medicine,
St. George's Hospital Medical School.

Dr. Bennett was once my Lecturer and during that time we put together some student notes. That those notes have found a new form in this book is witness to the commitment of the teaching staff at the Royal London Hospital and Prof Shah Ebrahim's and Dr. Bennett's enthusiasm for their subject. As I read through the manuscript I realised how little of the embryo remains in the adult form, and I congratulate them on the work they have done to make our subject more readily understandable by others.

The book is in three parts. The first part considers aspects of ageing as it impinges on the older person. The second reminds the reader of the roots of the specialty of geriatric medicine before moving on to explore the different presentation of disease in old age. The third examines the multi-disciplinary aspects of care of the older patient. Each section stands alone, and within each chapter is a little vignette which ends with the key points.

Although I must admit to bias, I don't think that it was just because of the complimentary things said about my contribution to the development of person-alised single room accommodation for the long stay patient, or because of my involvement with the early notes, that I liked the book. I think my reason for liking it was that it was easy to read and contained useful knowledge which you will not find in other books.

The book is complementary to textbooks of medicine. Disease sometimes presents classically in the aged person. But usually it presents in a more subtle way, and often comes disguised as social problems.

Shakespeare wrote about the seven ages of man, and no self-respecting ninety year old comes into hospital without at least seven things wrong with them. Illness in old age is a complex interweave of biological, psychological and environmental factors, which is why geriatric medicine is an appealing clinical speciality to practice.

Fascinating problems still wait to be solved. Amongst them are questions such as: Why do elderly people have a tendency to fall backwards after a period of bed rest? Is it because their anti-gravity muscles are disordered? Or is there a lesion in some yet to be discovered 'posturostat'? Viewed from the perception of youth old age may have little charm, but old people see ageing differently. Why is that? Why do women live longer than men? Is it all to do with the women being XX, or is there a more deep seated motivational factor that explains why women survive illness better than men. If so can men learn what it is and change their survival pattern? You won't find the answers to those questions in this book, but what you will find is the basic knowledge that will enable you to make a good attempt to tackle the practical problems of falling, confusion, immobility and incontinence.

Reading the book I thought of Richard Asher's essays in the book 'Talking Sense'. Three things brought it to mind. Firstly, his article 'Aren't I Lucky I Can Write' sums up my agonies in creative writing and leaves me with admiration of those who write books. Secondly, his article 'The Dangers of Bed Rest', quoted in this book, dramatically portrays the dangers of prolonged bed rest: reading it now one can see how much care of the chronic sick has advanced in the last fifty years. Thirdly, because this book, like the collection of his writings, contains considerable commonsense.

Geriatric medicine was not taught when I was an undergraduate. I studied at University College Hospital, and qualified in 1960. Two years later in the West Cameroons, West Africa, I was one of four doctors for a million people. Each of us had our own hospital. The next doctor was forty miles away. I knew what I was meant to do, but I did not know how to do it. But there were books and using them I struggled to be the obstetrician, paediatrician, physician, surgeon, public health doctor. Surprisingly the death rate went down!

In 1964 I returned to the United Kingdom and entered into geriatric medicine as an S.H.O. in a seaside town. There I was the fourth doctor in a geriatric department with 180 beds, 120 of which contained bed-bound patients, and I had no idea what I was meant to do. I knew I was meant to rehabilitate, but nobody had ever taught me how to do that. And there were few books about the special knowledge necessary to practise geriatric medicine.

Gradually, over the years, the truth dawned. You rehabilitate patients by changing the environments in which they are treated. You lower the beds and you raise the chairs. You remove the cot sides so the patients can get out of bed, and when they are out you dress them in their own clothes. Then you treat them with respect, and on ward rounds you watch them attempt to walk and you praise their every effort. Occasionally you give them an aid to assist them, but usually you just congratulate them on what they have achieved, for ninety per cent of rehabilitation is done with the mouth. Now, looking back, it all seems so simple, but it couldn't have seemed so simple when the attack on bed rest began.

The knowledge gained by doctors who struggled to introduce rehabilitation to the chronic sick wards underpins the specialty of geriatric medicine. From those pioneers we learned that the science of medicine has to be complemented by the art. This book will help you to do that and I wish it well.

Acknowledgements

We thank our colleagues at St George's Hospital Medical School, Nottingham University Medical School, The Royal Free Hospital School of Medicine, The Medical College of St Bartholomew's Hospital and the London Hospital Medical College who have contributed greatly to the concepts contained in this book. Our thanks also go to Miss Julianna Hayward for expert typing of the manuscript.

Dedication

We dedicate this book to our patients, their carers and the teams who look after them.

PART ONE
ESSENTIALS OF AGEING

1 AGEING: POPULATIONS, ORGANISMS AND CELLS

- Medical care versus social care
- Impairments, disabilities and handicaps
- Population ageing
- Rectangularization of survival
- Individual ageing
- Mechanisms of human ageing

Ageing is a developmental process, part of the cycle beginning at conception and ending with death. Ageing is not the same as disease, but diseases do become much more common among older people. This association of ageing and disease is the cause of much confusion about what is in store for us as we age, and it is a confusion that tends to affect doctors more

Table 1.1 The relationships between ageing and disease

| GETTING IN AND OUT OF BATH | Disease Process (e.g. Osteomalacia) | |
	Present	*Absent*
Unable	May be due to the disease	May be due to age-related decline in strength
Able	Occult disease	Healthy

than their patients. Patients complain to their doctors of pain and immobility only to be told that their problems are due to their age — which is seldom true.

Consider, for example, a patient who develops difficulty getting in and out of the bath. This may be due to a decline in the number of functioning muscle cells (ageing) leading to weakness. Alternatively it may be due to a disease affecting the peripheral nerves, a metabolic disease (e.g. diabetes or osteomalacia), or disease of large joints (e.g. osteoarthritis). This is demonstrated in Table 1.1.

MEDICAL CARE VERSUS SOCIAL CARE

In the example given above, a social model of care would lead to assessment of the problem and provision of a bath board and rails around the bath. A medical model would sort out disease from ageing, and attempt to treat any underlying disease process. A collaborative approach would lead to both treatment (in its widest sense) of any disease underlying the disability, and provision of any aids or lifestyle modifications to overcome the disability. Collaboration and teamwork are the hallmarks of health care of the elderly.

The medical model is often criticized for its preoccupation with diagnosis and drug treatment, for its focus on organ systems, and for its super-specialization. But the medical model has much to offer elderly people. Disease does become so much more common with increasing age and deserves to be diagnosed and treated. Despite much disease being chronic, degenerative and irreversible, much can be done for its disabling and handicapping consequences. However, the doctor is seldom able to combat disease consequences single-handedly. Teamwork is necessary, and the concept of diagnosis has to be extended to assessment, treatment becomes management, and prognosis becomes monitoring and evaluation of achievement of goals.

An exclusively social model, bypassing the question 'Is this problem due to disease or not?', is as inadequate for solving problems as a solely medical model. Collaboration is essential, and is best achieved through comprehensive services for elderly people.

IMPAIRMENTS, DISABILITIES AND HANDICAPS

Although these terms are often used interchangeably, they do have precise meanings that help us to understand what comprehensive care means.

Table 1.2 Definitions of impairment, disability and handicap

Impairment
Damage caused to a cell, organ or system by a disease process

Disability
Difficulty in carrying out tasks — such as activities of daily living, or driving a car — that are a consequence of the disease

Handicap
Effect the disease has on the lifestyle of the patient — the disadvantage caused by the disease

Some treatment may reduce *impairment*. For example, exercise against progressively increased resistance may increase muscle strength and joint flexibility in an arthritic joint. The measurement of muscle strength and joint range of movement would be the best indicators of success or failure.

Other treatments may have no effect whatsoever on the impairment caused by disease. For example, no amount of physiotherapy will reduce the amount of

brain damaged by a stroke. However, therapy may well reduce the time taken to get independently mobile again. In this case the correct measure of success is the reduction in *disability* (or more positively, increase in *mobility*).

With many diseases, neither the impairment nor the disability is affected by rehabilitation teamwork. This is not to say that useful management is impossible. Some patients are viewed as 'no-hopers' on an acute medical ward, but are transformed into 'major rehabilitation challenges' on a ward for health care of the elderly. There is no special magic in this, but simply a more realistic appraisal of the possibilities by the team, and a tendency to focus on *handicap* (or more positively, *lifestyle*).

It is vital that those involved in services for elderly people understand their contribution to the overall picture, and do not attempt to demonstrate the supremacy of their particular skills. The impairments, disabilities, and handicaps framework (summarized in Table 1.2) is a useful way of ensuring a comprehensive approach.

POPULATION AGEING

We are living in an ageing society, indicated by such phenomena as the greying of America, the rise of the Grey Panthers, and the growth of retirement and nursing homes. One of the major justifications for health care of the elderly is the increased numbers of elderly people. This is highlighted by the tremendous increase in the numbers of centenarians in the UK who received a birthday telegram from the Queen (see Fig. 1.1).

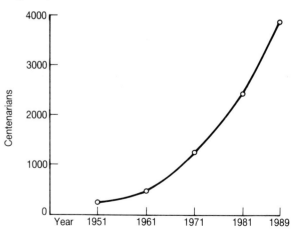

Figure 1.1 The dramatic increase in the number of centenarians in the UK

The spectacular population changes over the last century can be best understood by looking at developing countries now. The major factor that makes populations age is 'family planning' — reducing the number of babies born and increasing the maternal age at first birth. A willingness to use family planning methods depends on culture, education and religion, but with increased economic wealth a move to smaller families is inevitable. Prosperity is no longer measured by the size of the family. Declines in fertility have contributed to the speed at which ageing is occurring in developing countries, particularly in Asia.

Table 1.3 Expectation of life (in years) at birth and at age 60, in the period 1975–80

	At birth		At 60 years	
	M	F	M	F
Africa	47	50	13.4	14.7
East Asia	66	69	16.0	17.7
South Asia	50	51	13.8	14.8
North America	69	77	16.8	20.3
Latin America	60	64	15.1	16.9
Europe	69	75	16.7	19.5
USSR	65	74	15.8	19.2
Oceania	64	68	15.6	17.5

maternal and child health services (immunization, sanitation, clean water, promotion of breast feeding, better maternal nutrition), and in part due to socio-economic development. These improvements in infant health have also contributed to the dramatic increase in the rate of ageing of the population.

Another major variable in the ageing of populations is the falling death rate at older ages. Over the last century the world has — despite appearances — become a healthier place to live, and more of us are doing it for longer (see Table 1.3 and Fig. 1.2).

It is paradoxical that an ageing population is a consequence of living in a 'successful' society that ensures that babies do not die, that promotes the autonomy of women to control their fertility, and that has reduced the chances of death over the entire lifespan. The large numbers of elderly people are our heritage, and the rewards of socio-economic development. Turning back the clock to the turn of the century when old age was not a 'problem' is impossible, and countries where high fertility and infant mortality occur do not wish to stay at that point in development. A better understanding of ageing, removing the myths and stereotypes, and improving the health, social and economic lot of elderly people are keys to the solution.

Total population

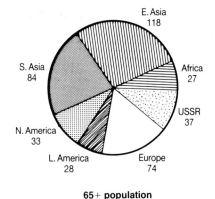

65+ population

Figure 1.2 World population expected in the year 2000 (in millions)

In developing countries the chances of dying in the first year of life are high; so high, that this infant mortality reduces the average expectation of life. If a baby gets through its first year of life, the risk of dying falls and its expectation of life rises quite dramatically. Many developing countries have enjoyed massive reductions in infant mortality, in part due to better

RECTANGULARIZATION OF SURVIVAL

Survival curves have changed in shape over the last few hundred years. This process has been called the 'rectangularization of survival' (see Fig. 1.3). One of the consequences of the increased chances of survival is that the average life expectancy begins to approach the maximum lifespan. The maximum lifespan is around 115 years, but the average expectation of life at

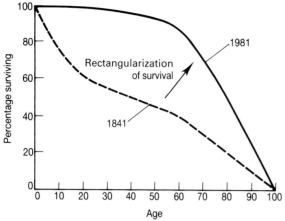

Figure 1.3 The rectangularization of survival: survival curves for 1841 and 1981

birth is around 80 years for women in the most successful countries (Japan, USA). Deaths, instead of being spread across a fairly long part of the human lifespan, are now compressed into a shorter time. This should mean that people are sicker for a shorter time as well, and in essence will tend to be healthier for longer.

This optimistic scenario for the next century may come true, but for the foreseeable future it is more likely that increased survival will be associated with increased risk of non life-threatening, but disabling chronic diseases. At present, the rectangularization of survival is associated with a far greater number of very old people which is producing an explosion of morbidity, and an increased pressure on health and social care resources.

INDIVIDUAL AGEING

We have become used to hearing how things change — usually for the worse — as we get older. Blood pressure goes up, hearing and vision get worse, bone density declines, intelligence declines, and so on. As humans grow and develop they reach a peak in physiological and anatomical capacity in their late teens, but subsequently capacity declines. It seems to matter little which type of capacity is considered: muscle strength, stamina, lung volume, kidney function and brain volume all show age-related declines.

Cross-sectional and longitudinal studies

There is a large trap for the unwary here. Most of the studies of age-related declines are not really studies of *ageing* at all. In fact they are studies of a number of young people, a number of middle-aged people, and a number of old and very old people, all examined at the same point in time. None of the subjects has aged at all *during* the study; they are simply of different ages at the time of the study. Such studies are cross-sectional 'snapshots', and we have to make some assumptions before we can accept that they are a good indication of true ageing changes.

The *first assumption* is that what is true now for 60-year-olds will be true for 50-year-olds in 10 years time. We have to believe that the effects of belonging to a group (or a cohort) of people born at around the same time, and living through a unique set of life experiences, are not relevant to the factor (e.g. blood pressure, brain volume) under study. However, the effects of belonging to a cohort have been extremely important over the last century. For example, women born at the turn of the century had far fewer chances for marriage than those born later, because of the First World War. Further, men who went to fight in that war, if they survived, were subsequently much more likely to die of lung cancer because of smoking habits acquired during the war. Cohort effects can be powerful, and are impossible to detect in a simple cross-sectional study.

The *second assumption* is that conducting the study at a particular point in time is irrelevant. It may seem unlikely that a cross-sectional study of changes in, say, muscle strength with age conducted in 1989 would come up with results different from one conducted in 1990. But over a period as short as five years, differences in the relationship between blood pressure and age *have* been found.

A *third assumption* is that older subjects are free from disease. For example, reductions in air flow with age may be due to changes in the elasticity of the lung, but inclusion of older people with chronic bronchitis will lead to much greater age-related reductions in air flow owing to the combined effects of age and disease.

Scientists continue to examine the effects of age by cross-sectional methods because they are generally much cheaper than cohort (follow-up or longitudinal) studies. Provided such studies give more or less the same answer, no harm is done. However, in the few cases where comparisons can be made between cross-sectional and cohort studies, the answers can be strikingly different.

Take, for example, performances on intelligence tests. The general conclusion of cross-sectional studies is that intelligence declines with age, which supports stereotyped images of confused old people. The cohort changes are strikingly different: far from getting more stupid over the years, people tend to improve on some aspects of intelligence and remain more or less the same on others, and decline in only a few areas (see Fig. 1.4).

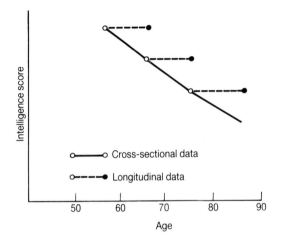

Figure 1.4 Changes in intelligence with age: cross-sectional and cohort studies compared

So why the difference? It probably arises out of a cohort effect. People born in 1920 had limited schooling and access to educational mass media like television and newspapers. People born in 1930 enjoyed better education. When studied cross-sectionally in 1990, those born in 1920 are 70 years old and do worse on the intelligence tests than the 60-year-olds born in 1930.

Describing true effects of ageing

Describing true ageing effects requires complicated studies of successive cohorts of people over long periods of time, or so-called 'cohort-sequential studies'. This is because a single cohort invariably experiences a unique set of circumstances thrown up by the era they live through (e.g. wars, economic depression) — period effects that have an impact at all ages. The task is to separate the effects of ageing from the effects of the era in which people age. This can only be done by studying a *succession* of cohorts to determine whether age-related changes are consistent across

each cohort. Very few such studies have been set up, so we usually have to make do with the information from cross-sectional studies. However, never take such information at face value: always ask, 'Could this be due to cohort or time-period effects?'

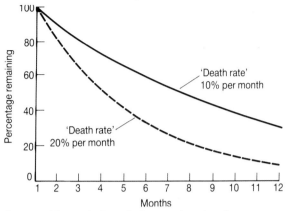

Figure 1.5 Theoretical survival curves for wine glasses

Statistically, ageing can be defined as 'facing an increased risk of death over time'. To see what this means, an analogy may help. If you take 1000 wine glasses and count how many 'survive' over a period of months, you would not be surprised if many of them 'died'. The death rate of the glasses can be calculated as the number broken divided by the number at the outset. However, a small adjustment has to be made for the fact that once a glass is broken it cannot be broken again, and must be removed from the denominator of the calculation for the 'death' rate. If this is done, a glass survival curve can be drawn, giving the percentage of glasses surviving at the end of each month (see Fig. 1.5). Now glasses do not age: their molecules contain no ability to replicate, they are inert. And yet a population of glasses appears to 'age', and has a survival curve. The key is that the rate of breakage of glasses is constant — there is a constant accident hazard that systematically removes glasses until they are all gone. Death rates of populations do not show a constant rate, but an ever increasing rate with increasing chronological age. This gives population survival curves their characteristic rectangular shape (Fig. 1.3). The point at which death rates start to rise can be viewed as the start of human ageing. It comes as a surprise to see how early in life this starts — in late teens or early twenties!

Many factors change as people get older. Some people get richer, most get poorer. Their homes age with them, often becoming hazardous. Social contacts and status within the family alter. These are called 'extrinsic factors', in contrast to intrinsic (or genetic) factors associated with ageing.

MECHANISMS OF HUMAN AGEING

Ageing has fascinated scientists, philosophers and poets for centuries. What is ageing? Why do we age? What is ageing for? How can we slow down or stop the process? These are weighty questions and need unravelling into smaller questions that are more easily tackled. An inherent difficulty in the study of ageing is that the findings from easy-to-study animal species (bacteria, paramecium, mice) are not directly transferable to humans.

Strehler's framework of ageing states that for a process to be truely due to ageing (rather than due to pathology) it must be universal, progressive, intrinsic and deleterious.

Cells get old and die just like the whole organism, but they do it at a more rapid rate. The cells of the epidermal layer of the skin shed themselves within a few days.

The red blood cell lives for about four months. Theories of ageing have to accommodate the following observations about ageing.

The Hayflick limit to cell division

The Hayflick limit is the number of cell divisions that human fibroblasts — connective tissue cells — grown in a cell culture can undergo before stopping. They stop after about 50 cell divisions. By contrast, many human cancer cells continue to replicate unchecked, and are called immortal.

Rate of DNA repair

DNA is damaged in the rough and tumble of cellular life, so DNA repair enzymes deal with the problems spontaneously. Species that are long-lived, such as humans and elephants, tend to have better DNA repair efficiency than short-lived species.

Increased autoimmune damage and reduction in protective immune responses

As people get older they become more prone to infections, such as pneumonia, and cell-mediated immunity to diseases like tuberculosis may wane, leading to a greater risk of disease. The occurrence of auto-antibody diseases (e.g. thyroid disease, pernicious anaemia, collagen-vascular diseases) is more common with age.

Accelerated ageing syndromes (progeria, Down's syndrome, diabetes)

The very rare inherited premature ageing, or progeria, syndromes lead to early death with many of the characteristics of very old people. The fibroblast cells of affected people demonstrate a reduced ability to replicate.

Increased cross-linking in DNA, collagen, proteins

Collagen fibres start to form rigid cross-linked sulphur bonds which interfere with connective tissue functions. In DNA, cross-links may form which are difficult to break, leading to errors in replication.

Enzyme, second messenger, accumulation of lipofuscin changes

Many cellular functions appear to change with increasing age. It is difficult to know which are prime forces in ageing, and which are merely consequences of more fundamental changes.

Energy use per kg per lifetime between different species

With the exception of humans, the rate at which different species use energy is roughly similar when allowance is made for body weight. Mice that are starved live longer than those fed at will.

Damage theories

The damage theories of cellular ageing are strongly supported by work on DNA repair enzymes and free radicals. Free radicals are oxidants, electron donors, produced as a byproduct of metabolism, and have an extra free electron. They are unstable, and when they combine with cell membranes lead to damage, producing lipid peroxides and aldehydes which cause increased cross-linking in proteins and DNA. Many enzyme systems are devoted to combating the adverse effects of free radicals. Antioxidants include vitamins C and E and selenium, and are often included in proprietary 'anti-ageing' drugs. There is no evidence that these drugs work.

The damage and toxic accumulation theories have been described as the 'clinker' theory, perhaps after the deposit that is found in the grate of an open fire or from its American usage as a term for a mistake or error. Somatic mutation caused by radiation exposure is another variant of the error theories, but is now discounted as the levels of radiation would have to be far too high to explain ageing changes.

Programmed ageing: genetic theories

Programme theories state that ageing is developmentally controlled. The whole process from conception, differentiation, growth and senescence is under a regulatory gene complex.

But if ageing is under genetic control, and we are programmed to age, what possible evolutionary advantage could it hold for us as individuals or as a species? After the reproductive phase of the lifespan it might be thought that the genome had done its job (which is in essence to reproduce itself), and was of no further use. Evolutionary selection of longevity genes would be of no advantage. Indeed salmon, for example, do die immediately after the reproductive phase, and this is a programmed self-destruction.

However, it is possible that longevity genes are linked with characteristics that make us more resistant to disease, or make us more ingenious, and that ageing is simply an unfortunate by-product of advantages reaped earlier in life. At a species level, the advantages of elders for social organization and repositories of knowledge may have outweighed their physical disadvantages, allowing the older men continued access to women as the means for ensuring the survival of their genes.

The programmed ageing theories and the damage theories can be brought together. It is possible that the regulation of DNA repair mechanisms, of antioxidants and of immunological mechanisms is under programmed genetic control. There is evidence that the major histocompatability system in the mouse is associated with both immunological competence and with longevity. The comparable HLA system in humans is associated with several autoimmune disease processes and in Japanese is associated with survival until over 90 years of age.

Theories of ageing are summarized in Table 1.4.

Table 1.4 Theories of ageing: a summary

Genetic–molecular theories
1. Codon restriction: accuracy of DNA–mRNA impaired
2. Error theories: accuracy of mRNA–proteins impaired
3. Gene regulation: post-reproductive changes in gene expression
4. Somatic mutation: radiation damage to DNA

Cellular theories
1. Wear and tear: with use the body wears out and dies
2. Age pigment: lipofuscin deposition as a primary cause of ageing
3. Free-radicals: lead to cell damage and thus ageing
4. Cross-linking: increased cross-linkage leading to irreversible damage to DNA and enzymes

System level theories
1. Neuro-endocrine control: a biological clock controls development through neural and hormonal mechanisms
2. Immune control: thymus gland as an 'immunological clock' leading to cell destruction due to failure to recognize self

Theories of ageing: so what?

Unravelling the mystery of why we age will inevitably preoccupy some scientists as an end in itself. The more exciting possibilities lie in understanding how to alter the expression of DNA, to reverse some of the adverse effects of ageing. At the individual level it may be possible to reduce the rate at which some organ systems decline by active interventions such as physical exercise. At the population level, the forecasting of changes in the future should allow us time to develop health and social policy. Such policies should allow us to alleviate some of the adverse consequences of an ageing population, and use some of the positive benefits of having large numbers of experienced senior citizens.

Key Points

- Population ageing is the result of reductions in infant mortality and fertility, and reduction in mortality at older ages. These changes are consequences of 'successful' societies with high levels of socio-economic development.
- Organ systems of individuals age at different rates, but all show decline starting in early adult life.
- Cross-sectional studies of the effects of ageing may hide changes associated with the cohort studied and the time period in which the study is conducted.
- Cellular ageing may be due to damage to DNA, and cellular proteins which may be regulated

genetically, bringing together the damage and genetic theories of ageing.

FURTHER READING

Clarke CA. Centenarians and the ultimate age attainable by man. *Nutrition Bulletin* 1984; **13**:132–140.

Coni N, Davison W, Webster S. *Ageing: The Facts.* Oxford University Press, Oxford, 1984.

Comfort A. *The Biology of Senescence,* 3rd edn. Elsevier. New York, 1979.

Fries JF, Green LW, Levine S. Health promotion and the compression of morbidity. *Lancet* 1989; **i**:481–483.

Takata H, Suzuki M, Ishii T, Sekiguchi S, Iri H. Influence of major histocompatability complex region genes on human longevity among Okinawan-Japanese centenarians and nonagenarians. *Lancet* 1987; **ii**:824–826.

Timiras PS (ed.). *Physiological Basis of Aging and Geriatrics.* Macmillan, London, 1988.

2 AGEING SKIN

- Epidermis and dermis
- Ultraviolet light
- Transparent skin
- Senile purpura
- Hair
- Pruritus
- Leg ulcers
- Anti-ageing measures

The generally held view is that as skin ages it normally develops characteristic physiological signs such as wrinkles, pigment alteration and thinning. It is now known that these are not normal ageing effects but pathological changes due mainly to ultraviolet light exposure. Obviously some conditions will occur as a result of unavoidable environmental exposure, genetics, and the effects of disease, but normal ageing produces surprisingly few skin changes. Exposure to sunlight, however, produces very deleterious effects. Some of the pathological conditions are keratoses, squamous cell carcinomas, basal cell carcinomas and malignant melanoma. Less life-threatening effects include wrinkling and hyper- and hypopigmentation. Thus there is very little evidence that the skin 'ages' apart from the effects of genetics, environment and disease.

EPIDERMIS AND DERMIS

Changes to the epidermis are minimal and subtle. The exposed skin may be slightly thicker and oxygen consumption may be slightly decreased. Metabolic processes appear unchanged.

In the dermis, changes in collagen are qualitative more than quantitative. There is some decrease in thickness especially in light-exposed skin, but the main changes include an increase in the cross-links on the collagen with some deterioration in fibre organization. The flexibility of the skin is due to the dermal collagen and there is minor deterioration with age. However, it is very marked in the pathological state known as the 'transparent skin syndrome' (see below).

ULTRAVIOLET (UV) LIGHT

The dangerous components of UV light are the shorter wavelengths, the effects being initially erythema ('sunburn'), increased thickness of the stratum corneum and increased melanocytes (hence a 'suntan'). Repeated exposure, especially with burning, results in pathological effects, including the skin cancers. This is important because fashionable advertising tells us that 'brown is beautiful' and that suntans are healthy. The side effects of accelerated skin ageing and the potential dangers are not mentioned.

Early pathological changes include yellowing and the formation of wrinkles (though heavy wrinkles probably have a genetic component). A few people develop de-pigmentation and obvious superficial 'broken' blood vessels — telangiectasia. The back of the hands as well as the face can develop keratotic nodules. The skin around the eyes may show yellow plaques — Dubreuilh's elastoma. The thick, deeply lined 'crazy paving' skin on the back of sun-exposed necks has the wonderful name of cutis rhomboidalis nuchae of Jadassohn!

Other sun-induced changes include keratoacanthoma, basal cell carcinoma and squamous cell carcinoma. The most dangerous is the malignant melanoma now becoming so common in Australia — doctors have been doing 'rounds' on the beaches, examining people and giving advice.

Very little is known about skin changes with age in the black population.

TRANSPARENT SKIN

Some individuals have skin like tissue paper, especially on the backs of the hands and forearms (see

Figure 2.1 Transparent skin syndrome

Fig. 2.1). This is probably a pathological condition and not an ageing process. The skin is loose and wrinkled and the underlying structures are seen easily. This type of skin has very poor elastic (i.e. tensile) properties. Histologically there is a thin dermis.

Interestingly the condition is associated with osteoporosis and hence collagen abnormalities may

be implicated. The skin 'tears' easily and is difficult to suture; it also bleeds and bruises easily. A similar finding is found in patients who have taken steroids ('steroid atrophy') and in patients with rheumatoid arthritis.

Transparent skin may also have white pseudoscars (thought to be due to episodes of minor trauma) and the skin has an increased tendency to senile purpura (see below).

The condition could possibly be related to other lax-skin conditions which are increasingly being diagnosed in non-pure forms.

SENILE PURPURA

Many elderly people develop bruising, especially over the hands and arms, without having the full-blown transparent skin syndrome. It is presumed that they have less elastic collagen and hence blood vessels are less well tethered and are more easily ruptured by minor trauma. The purpura stays longer because reabsorption is much slower. Other vascular changes include the appearance of a few spider naevi and an occasional splinter haemorrhage under the fingernails (traumatic in origin). The most common skin lesion noted is the small red Campbell de Morgan spot, a benign lesion seen most often on the trunk and abdomen.

HAIR

Grey hair is genetically determined (autosomal dominant) and is far less worrying for the individual than the loss of hair (again genetically determined in men). Both men and women lose their hair with age; men simply lose it sooner, faster and more comprehensively! Male vanity and the media have determined that enormous sums are being spent to stop and reverse this most benign of ageing processes.

PRURITUS

This is so common in the elderly that the term 'senile pruritus' is well known. Again, pathology rather than normal ageing is more important in the aetiology, diagnosis and treatment (see Table 2.1).

Table 2.1 Common causes of pruritus in the elderly

Drugs

Blood disorders (e.g. polycythaemia rubra vera, anaemia)

Malignant disease (e.g. lymphomas)

Liver and kidney disease (esp. with jaundice and uraemia)

Dryness (exacerbated by washing, detergent residues in clothes, temperature)

Infestations (scabies, lice)

Skin disorders (eczema, lichen planus, pre-pemphigoid)

Incontinence (effects of urine and faeces)

Figure 2.2 Venous leg ulcer

LEG ULCERS

It is estimated that there are 100 000 people with active leg ulcers in the UK and that the majority occur in the elderly. Approximately 50 per cent of leg ulcers are due to venous stasis (see Fig. 2.2), 10 per cent to arterial disease and 30–40 per cent are mixed.

All patients with a leg ulcer need a full clerking, asking especially about pregnancies, venous thromboses and current drugs. Unusual causes need to be considered — is the ulcer malignant, arteritic or secondary to the side-effects of drugs?

If oedema is present the cause should be ascertained, as well as a complete history concerning mobility and whether the person sleeps in bed or in a chair with feet resting on a low and ineffective stool (this situation has often resulted from the effects of the swelling causing relative or absolute immobility). Salt and water retention with non-steroidal preparations can result in leg oedema.

Examination should include feeling for pulses and the measurement of ankle blood pressure using a Doppler meter to determine whether the arterial circulation is adequate. The ulcer needs to be accurately described including any surrounding haemosiderin (evidence of regular small thromboses) and eczema. The size needs to be measured, which can be done using exposed x-ray film and an indelible marker.

The presence of significant oedema requires a few days of bed-rest (with diuretics only if there are signs of heart failure). The ulcer should be cleaned with saline and systemic antibiotics used only if there is definite evidence of cellulitis. The effect of bed-rest can be dramatic, but the ulcer itself can be painful and analgesics should be given.

The correct management of venous ulcers (after Doppler assessment to exclude arterial insufficiency) is pressure bandaging. This has to be effective, and so the type of bandage, its application and the role of exercise and elevation require a good level of skill and communication. Healing rates of up to 90 per cent can be obtained. In selected cases surgery to incompetent veins is helpful.

An *arterial component* to the ulcer is more common in the elderly (hence the need for pressure measurement), and the wrong use of pressure bandaging on an arterial ulcer can be disastrous. Arterial ulcers can be difficult to heal. The patient may have evidence of vascular disease elsewhere. Smoking is heavily implicated and benefit can still be obtained by stopping even at this late stage.

Attention to detail (not elevating the foot, taking care of the surrounding skin with soft material and pressure area care) means that the ulcers may heal, but quite slowly. Large vessel disease may benefit from vascular surgery intervention and an opinion should be sought. Patients with diabetes mellitus get pressure ulcers on the feet very easily (secondary to the neuropathy) and they also suffer from small vessel-disease. Sadly some ischaemic foot ulcers require amputation to alleviate pain and infection.

ANTI-AGEING MEASURES

Because the superficial effects of 'ageing' are so visible, and especially in a youth-obsessed culture, it is not surprising that a whole industry has developed to keep people 'looking younger'. More could be achieved simply by avoiding sunlight.

Most creams are useless apart from their camouflage effect. However, isotretinoin (a vitamin A derivative used to treat severe acne) does cause 'peeling' in normal skin, so erasing the finest of the wrinkles. More dramatic is the use of plastic surgery, whereby 'face-lifts' are becoming increasingly popular. People should be warned, however, that repeat procedures may lead to the umbilicus becoming an unusual beauty-spot on the chin!

KEY POINTS

- Normal physiological ageing produces few skin changes.
- The pathological effects of ultraviolet light produce wrinkles, thin/transparent skin, pigmentation changes and benign and malignant tumours.
- Senile purpura is common and is due to poor blood vessel tethering.
- Grey hair is genetically determined and occurs to some degree in both sexes.

- Approximately 50 per cent of leg ulcers are due to venous stasis, 10 per cent to arterial disease and 40 per cent mixed.
- Assessment of leg ulcers includes Doppler measurement and measurement (by tracing) of size.
- To avoid 'ageing' changes and cosmetic surgeons — do not sunbathe!

FURTHER READING

Fenske NA, Lober CW. Structural and functional changes of normal ageing skin. *J Am Acad Dermatol* 1986; **15**:571–585.

Strehler BL (ed.). *Advances in Gerontological Research*, vols 1 and 2. Academic Press, New York, 1964 and 1967.

3 THE AGEING EYE

- Appearance
- Anterior chamber
- Presbyopia
- Cataract
- Other ageing effects
- Acute and chronic visual loss

Apart from being the windows to the soul, the eyes of elderly people are interesting both in health and disease. The transition from physiological (age-related) to pathological (disease-related) change can be indistinct. In normal ageing there may be some loss of visual acuity and a greater propensity to cataract formation. Other changes, including most of the 'ageing changes' reported, are in fact pathological.

APPEARANCE

Characteristically the eyes are sunken as a result of loss of periorbital fat; this may be severe enough to cause drooping of the upper lid (ptosis) and redundant skin at the lateral borders. The loss of fat can also cause the lower eyelid to curl in (entropion) and irritate the cornea, causing redness and watering (epiphora). A simple stop-gap measure is to apply tape just below the eyelid and pull it down slightly using the adhesive effect of the tape on the cheek: this will suffice until an expert opinion can be sought and a minor surgical procedure performed if necessary. The laxity also enables the eyelid to fall outwards slightly (ectropion); again this can lead to epiphora and subsequent inflammation and conjunctivitis.

A whitish circle around the iris (arcus senilis, or gerontoxon) is seen in some elderly people, but as this is a lipid infiltrate in the periphery of the cornea it is probably not a true ageing process. It is initially comma-like at the top and bottom but eventually extends around until a dense white border results. A full arcus in a comparatively young person may indicate a lipid abnormality and premature ischaemic heart disease.

ANTERIOR CHAMBER

Numerous factors contribute to the anterior chamber becoming more shallow as we age. The lens especially becomes thicker and the size and shape of the eyeball changes. This can be clinically significant in the condition known as angle-closure glaucoma (see Fig.

3.1), when the iris blocks the fluid-filtering mechanism and the intraocular pressure rises acutely usually causing severe pain, vomiting and blurred vision. The condition can present however, as an acute confusional state or even as an 'acute abdomen' (owing to vomiting and collapse). Urgent diagnosis and referral to a specialist is required, and treatment may be medical (the use of drugs such as pilocarpine) or surgical.

condition is, however, familial and close relatives (including children) should be screened.

The pupillary diameter decreases with advancing age and the iris becomes more fibrous. There is thus a reduced response to accommodation and reduced light access. This means that, because of slower dark adaptation, additional illuminating light is needed. It has been estimated that the eye needs to double the illumination approximately every 13 years to maintain

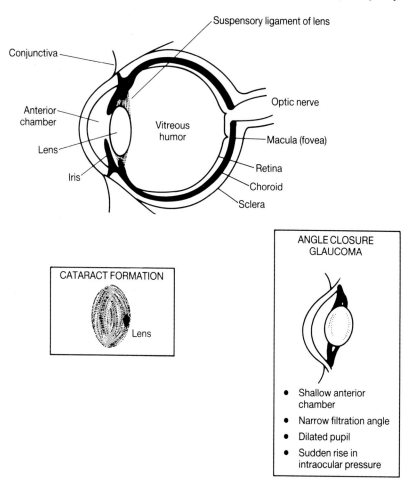

Figure 3.1 The eye and some age-related changes

Open-angle glaucoma is due to a much slower rise in the intraocular pressure (secondary to abnormal drainage of aqueous humor). Vision is gradually lost; 'tunnel vision' results and help may only be sought when this too is compromised. A routine examination may pick up pathological cupping of the optic disc, abnormal field defects or raised intraocular pressure. Treatment is again either medical or surgical. The

recognition in subdued light. Typical room lighting is around 150–200 watts, whereas, for optimal vision, elderly people require around 400 watts.

PRESBYOPIA

The crystalline lens (see Fig. 3.1) is unique in that, as we age, new lens fibres are laid down *over* the old (like layers of an onion skin). This results in the lens not only getting bigger, but it also becomes more dense and rigid. Focusing is achieved by relaxation of the suspensory ligament by the action of the ciliary muscle. The increased rigidity means, however, that the lens can no longer alter its shape sufficiently to become convex enough to allow adequate focusing. The power of the lens also reduces with age so that clarity for near objects is only achieved by increasing the focal length (i.e. by holding the object further away). Eventually one's arms are no longer long enough and corrective lenses are needed!

CATARACT

The increase in the layers around the lens is progressive and causes central compression. The middle becomes hard (nuclear sclerosis) and increasingly opaque. This phenomenon appears to be universal, making the eventual cataract formation a true ageing rather than pathological event. The posterior pole of the lens is a common site for this initial sclerosis; here it acts as a visual plug and, with the added problem of the smaller pupil, can cause an incapacitating loss of vision. Peripheral (cartwheel) cataracts may be initially less disabling, but eventually they cause light dispersal and can make vision impossible in bright light. Hence a lot of elderly people with these early cataracts wear peaked caps or shade bright lights to decrease this effect.

The metabolic changes within the lens are receiving considerable attention as possible markers of disease and as preventive pathways. There is a reduction in general metabolic activity with age but in cataract sufferers there is a marked decrease in the tripeptide glutathione (present in high concentrations in the normal lens). Soluble proteins are reduced and may have been changed into insoluble complexes or leaked out. Diabetics are extremely prone to cataract formation and in this condition the lens concentration and metabolism of sorbitol is markedly abnormal.

Much can be done to help in the management of the cataract affected elderly person. It is preferable to arrange reading lights to shine over the shoulder on to the page, thus ensuring the pupils are somewhat shaded and hence more dilated. Myopia should be corrected and pressures checked which will permit the pupils to be dilated (by drugs) to get light around a central or polar opacity. The increased risk of retinal detachment and glaucoma means that unilateral or second eye cataracts are not usually removed. Cataracts are removed surgically when poor vision interferes with normal activities. The operation can be done under local anaesthetic in selected cases. Postoperative contact lenses are not too successful in the more frail patient and spectacles with corrective lenses are more commonly used. Unfortunately the corrective aphakic lenses produce spherical aberrations which cause straight lines (such as the edges of a doorway) to appear curved. They also produce the jack-in-the-box effect whereby, on walking through doorways or confined spaces, the edges suddenly disappear only to reappear in a startling manner. Increasingly, lens implantation at the time of surgery is used with benefit.

OTHER AGEING EFFECTS

Vitreous opacities (floaters) result from degeneration of the vitreous body. They are common and unimportant but a sudden 'shower' may indicate a retinal detachment. Common fundal changes include drusen (pale patches) and senile macular degeneration (a dark mottled appearance around the macula). Macular degeneration is accompanied by decreased visual acuity, the only help being lenses with increased magnification. The use of bifocal spectacles to correct lens abnormalities is becoming increasingly popular. One hidden danger, especially in the elderly, is that depth perception is altered and falls can result, especially on stairs.

ACUTE AND CHRONIC VISUAL LOSS

Visual loss is a comparatively common symptom in elderly people. It can for convenience be subdivided into acute and chronic onset as in Table 3.1.

Causes of acute onset include retinal detachment (owing to the formation of a retinal hole and accompanied by flashes of light prior to loss of vision) and vascular conditions. Temporary loss of vision (amaurosis fugax) is usually secondary to platelet emboli formation. Total loss of vision is due to central retinal artery occlusion and is usually permanent. The cause of amaurosis fugax (i.e. the origin of the emboli) should be sought and treated. Retinal vein occlusion is more common and the clinical presentation is dependent on the nearness to the macula.

Table 3.1 Acute and chronic loss of vision

Acute onset
Retinal detachment
Vascular causes (central retinal artery/vein thrombosis)
Angle-closure glaucoma

Chronic onset
Cataract
Macular degeneration
Open-angle glaucoma
Diabetic retinopathy

Chronic onset loss of vision is most commonly caused by macular degeneration. In this condition hyaline deposits (drusen) occur on Bruchs membrane causing adhesions and impairing the blood supply, eventually causing loss of vision. For most patients there is no treatment apart from the use of magnifying aids.

Key points

- Altered fat distribution around the eyes can result in ptosis, entropion and ectropion.
- Acute angle-closure glaucoma requires urgent medical attention.
- Open-angle glaucoma causes gradual visual loss and is familial.
- The crystalline nature of the lens causes it to become dense and rigid, affecting focusing.
- Central lens compression leads to opaqueness and hence cataract formation.
- Macular degeneration is accompanied by decreased visual acuity, which can be helped by magnifying lenses.
- Visual loss may be of acute or chronic onset.
- Acute causes of visual loss include retinal detachment, central retinal artery thrombosis and acute angle-closure glaucoma.
- Chronic onset causes of visual loss include cataract, macular degeneration, open-angle glaucoma and diabetic retinopathy.

FURTHER READING

Cullinan T. *Visual Disability in the Elderly.* Croom Helm, London, 1986.
Graham P. The eye. In: Pathy MSJ (ed.), *Principles and Practice of Geriatric Medicine.* John Wiley, Chichester, 1985.
Wheale RA. *The Ageing Eye.* HK Lewis, London, 1963.

4 THE AGEING EAR

- Presbycusis
- Other changes
- Audiograms
- Hearing aids
- Communication with hearing-impaired people

Hearing impairment is extremely common in old age, with over half of those over 75 years having a hearing problem. The commonest cause of hearing loss with age (**presbycusis**) is due to an age-related decline in the ability to perceive tones above 2000 Hz. Speech frequencies are in the range 500 to 6000 Hz, with consonants tending to have higher frequencies than vowel sounds. Since much of the sense of speech is embodied in the consonants, high tone loss has a disproportionate effect on the ability to understand normal speech.

PRESBYCUSIS

Presbycusis is a **sensori-neural** form of deafness, meaning that it is caused by degeneration of the cochlea and its neurones, rather than **conductive** deafness which is due to problems with the middle or external ear (see Fig. 4.1). The underlying reasons for presbycusis are not known, but the process is progressive, bilateral and starts from about the age of 40. It is likely that genetic factors are involved in the occurrence of presbycusis: black men are less likely to suffer than white men, even if they have had heavy exposure to industrial noise.

OTHER CHANGES

The *external ear* is a frequent cause of problems. The skin of the meatus contains sebaceous and cerumen glands, which secrete wax. With age, the number and activity of these glands decline, leading to a reduction in skin moisture and a tendency to produce dry, impacted ear wax. These changes may also lead to itchiness in the ear, another common complaint, which can be aggravated by attempts to relieve the itch with hairpins or cotton-wool buds, leading to an itch–scratch–itch cycle.

In the *middle ear*, the conduction of sound from the ear drum to the cochlea is achieved through an intricate arrangement of the three bones, malleus, incus and stapes. With age, changes occur in the articular cartilage of these bones similar to those seen in larger arthritic joints (calcification in the joint capsule, reduction in the joint space, fraying of the

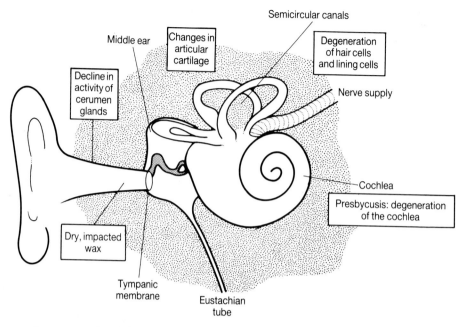

Figure 4.1 The ear and some age-related changes

joint cartilage). However, these changes do not seem to contribute to any conductive hearing loss.

In addition to presbycusis, the *inner ear* is affected by many disease processes that are commoner with age (vascular insufficiency, autoimmune diseases, neoplasms, Meniérè's disease, and drug-induced damage). The inner ear also serves in the control of balance, through the semicircular canals — the labyrinth. Like the cochlea, the labyrinth also suffers an age-related degeneration of its lining cells, its sensitive hair cells, and nerve fibres. While dizziness is a common symptom, it is seldom due to disease or ageing of the inner ear. Vertigo, the sensation of rotation, may be caused by many disease processes, but a condition called **benign paroxysmal positional vertigo** (in other words, vertigo occurring from time to time, and precipitated by the position of the head) may be caused by age-related degeneration of the labyrinth.

AUDIOGRAMS

Volume of noise is measured in decibels (dB), on a logarithmic scale. Speech ranges from less than 25 dB (a whisper), through 40–60 dB (normal speech), to 80 dB and above (shouting).

In testing hearing, a pure-tone audiogram presents sounds at a succession of frequencies (e.g. 250 Hz

through to 8000 Hz). At each frequency, the tone is made progressively louder until it is registered by the subject. Loss of up to 20 dB is considered within the normal range. Loss of hearing begins to be apparent when 30–40 dB is lost (see Fig. 4.2).

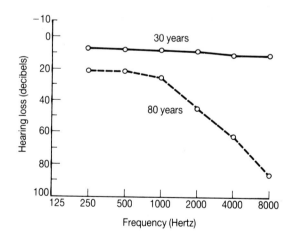

Figure 4.2 Presbycusis as demonstrated by two typical audiograms

In addition to the measurement of the response to pure tones, patients are asked to discriminate single-syllable words at normal volumes and the effects of amplification are measured. Those who do better with amplification will usually benefit from a hearing aid.

HEARING AIDS

It is important that the patient with hearing loss is a full partner in discussing management. If the patient has unrealistic expectations of what a hearing aid will offer, disappointment will be inevitable, and the aid will not be used. For every patient — and family — time will be required for counselling and review.

Volume control

Battery compartment

Ear mould

Off

Telecoil

Microphone = On

Microphone

Figure 4.3 Behind-the-ear hearing aid

A basic hearing aid amplifies sound; but as technology improves, aids are becoming smaller, more specific for speech frequencies, and some have noise-suppression units to aid speech discrimination in noisy environments. It is worth becoming familiar with the controls of aids and with simple maintenance: cleaning, changing batteries, reassembling (see Fig. 4.3).

COMMUNICATION WITH HEARING IMPAIRED PEOPLE

Shouting does not help, and may reduce the ability of a deaf person to understand. However, increasing the volume of speech a little is useful, and widely practised. The other keys to better communication are shown in Table 4.1.

Hearing impairment has powerful psychosocial

Table 4.1 Better communication with hearing-impaired people

1. Get the attention of the person
2. Ensure you face the person at the same level
3. Sit in a good light
4. Avoid eating or touching your mouth while speaking
5. Speak towards the better ear at a distance of up to 1 metre
6. Reduce background noise to the minimum
7. Speak slowly and clearly
8. If the person has a hearing aid, switch it on
9. If the person does not have an aid, speak loudly or use a portable amplifier or speaking tube

effects. It is a potent risk factor for depressive illness and also leads to withdrawal from social occasions. Early recognition and treatment of hearing problems is essential to reduce these all too common consequences.

Key points

- Loss of hearing in older people is most often due to presbycusis, a degeneration of the cochlea.
- Speech ranges from 25 dB (a whisper) to above 80 dB (shouting). Loss of hearing is apparent when 30-40 dB are lost.
- Provision of a hearing aid (which is an amplifier) requires careful counselling and review.
- Communication is aided by raising your voice (but not shouting), obtaining attention, sitting face to face, reducing background noise, and speaking slowly and clearly.
- Hearing impairment has powerful psychosocial effects, leading to isolation and depression, particularly if left untreated.

FURTHER READING

Han SS, Coons DH (eds). *Special Senses in Ageing.* Institute of Gerontology, University of Michegan, Ann Arbor, 1979.

Hinchcliffe R. *Hearing and Balance in the Elderly.* Churchill Livingstone, Edinburgh, 1983.

5 THE AGEING KIDNEY

- Age changes
- Impaired homeostasis
- Abnormalities of urea
- Electrolytes
- Problems with drugs

The kidney consists of millions of nephrons, each made up of a glomerulus (a filter with pores too small to let through simple proteins like albumen), a proximal tubule, a loop of Henle, and a distal tubule (see Fig. 5.1). The tubules and loop are responsible for the control of salt, water and acid–base balance. The proximal tubule carries out most of the active reabsorption and excretion processes that are energy- and enzyme-dependent. The loop of Henle and distal tubule produce the countercurrent multiplier effect that leads to urine concentration, regulated by the effects of antidiuretic hormone (ADH) and aldosterone.

AGE CHANGES

With increasing age the kidneys become smaller. A kidney in young adult life weighs about 400 g, but by the age of 90 it has shrunk to less than 300 g. Even more dramatic is the fall in the number of nephrons, of which half are lost between the ages of 40 and 70 years. The rate at which the glomeruli filter fluid — the glomerular filtration rate — also falls from 140 ml/minute/1.73 m² in mid-adult life by 8 ml/minute/1.73 m² for each decade. This rate of reduction in glomerular filtration is accelerated in people with high blood pressure.

However, simply losing nephrons does not lead to any problems as young people are capable of surviving perfectly well with only a single kidney. Indeed, a lone young kidney will hypertrophy as a compensatory change, although this does not occur in old age.

Renal blood flow also falls disproportionately to the reduction in renal size, and is most marked in the renal cortex. The glomerular basement membrane also changes, becoming more permeable, and more likely to let proteins through. In some glomeruli degenerative changes occur leading to sclerosis. These changes contribute to the reduction in surface area available for filtration, and explain the reduced glomerular filtration rate.

IMPAIRED HOMEOSTASIS

The renal changes are of no great significance in themselves, but they dramatically alter the ability of

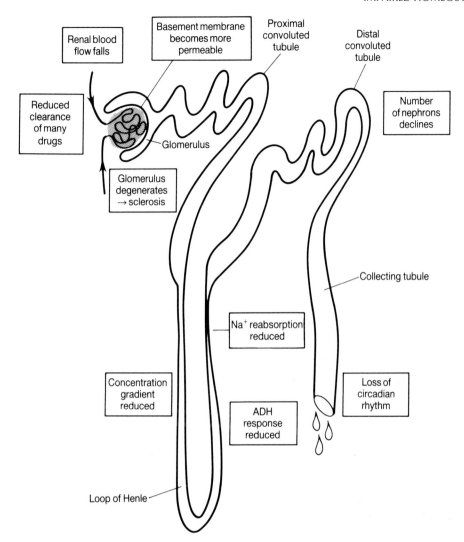

Figure 5.1 A nephron and some age-related changes

the body to compensate for external changes — to maintain homeostasis. For example, if salt is removed from the diet, the kidney will compensate by removing as much sodium as possible from the urine to achieve sodium balance. In young people this takes place twice as fast as it does in older people. The problem for older people is probably in the ascending limb of the loop of Henle where the ability to reabsorb sodium is greatly reduced. This in turn reduces the efficiency of the countercurrent multiplier system that concentrates urine, leading to a less efficient response to water depletion.

When faced with lack of water elderly people tend to produce more urine, and less concentrated urine than younger people. It is probable that elderly people, like patients with chronic renal failure, have to produce a finite volume of urine to ensure that the reduced number of nephrons are capable of dealing with the solute load. The renal blood flow to the medulla of the kidney is well preserved with age, whereas the cortical supply falls. It is possible that this relatively greater medullary flow washes away the normal concentration gradient.

The release of antidiuretic hormone is affected by ageing. If hypertonic saline is infused into a healthy elderly person, the expected increase in plasma ADH which normally leads to conservation of water is exaggerated. However, the effects of dehydration and moving from lying to standing, which also provoke an ADH response, are blunted in many elderly people.

Recent studies have demonstrated a loss of the circadian rhythms of urine excretion in elderly people, which may explain the need to get up at night to urinate.

ABNORMALITIES OF UREA

It is common for routine blood chemistry results to be reported as abnormal. It is as well to remember that the laboratory 'normal range' is usually based on data from young adults. It is also a statistical normal range; in other words, 95 per cent of healthy subjects will lie within the upper and lower limits. This also means that 5 per cent of healthy subjects will be outside the normal range.

Blood urea concentrations are often raised, particularly among hospital in-patients. This is usually due to dehydration, diuretic therapy, or both. The serum creatinine is usually within the normal range because muscle mass falls with increasing age.

ELECTROLYTES

A low plasma sodium concentration (hyponatraemia) is often a source of worry. Up to a quarter of all elderly patients admitted to hospital are hyponatraemic. It is necessary to decide whether the patient is volume-depleted, volume-expanded, or about normal. Volume depletion is common in patients on diuretic therapy that is aggressive and in those suffering with dehydration. Volume expansion occurs typically in congestive cardiac failure. The mechanisms to consider are the decreased ability to excrete water, water intoxication with concurrent diuretic therapy, and increased (inappropriate) ADH secretion. It is essential to measure the plasma osmolality to decide whether the patient is truly short of sodium, and therefore hypo-osmolar. If the patient has high levels of plasma lipids or proteins, the plasma sodium may be low (a pseudo-hyponatraemia), which does not imply any problem of salt and water balance.

High plasma sodium concentrations occur because of loss of body water (at a greater rate than loss of sodium), inadequate water intake, or increased sodium intake. Elderly people may not recognize that they are thirsty, leading to severe dehydration and hypernatraemia. This is very common amongst demented institutionalized patients.

PROBLEMS WITH DRUGS

Many drugs are excreted by the kidneys. Examples are digoxin, aminoglycoside antibiotics, oral hypoglycaemics, non-steroidal anti-inflammatory drugs, and anticholinergics. Reduced renal clearance of such drugs means that doses have to be reduced to avoid toxicity.

Diuretics are amongst the most commonly prescribed medications for elderly people, but given the precarious state of the ageing kidney they are often the cause of iatrogenic admissions to hospital with severe dehydration and electrolyte imbalance. Tetracyclines should also be avoided in old people as they have a catabolic effect which raises blood urea, and they may be nephrotoxic. Non-steroidal anti-inflammatory drugs in high dose may lead to renal failure; anticholinergics to acute confusional states; nitrofurantoin to a neuropathy; and aminoglycoside antibiotics to deafness and renal failure.

Key points

- Renal function declines with age. Approximately half the nephrons are lost between the ages of 30 and 70 years.
- Reduction in renal function leads to impaired homeostasis, making older people much more vulnerable to the effects of dehydration and water overload.
- Circadian rhythms of water excretion are lost, leading to nocturia.
- Many drugs are excreted by the kidney, and usual adult doses may lead to drug toxicity.

FURTHER READING

Kirkland JL, Lye M, Levy DW, Banerjee AK. Patterns of urine flow and electrolyte excretion in healthy elderly people. *Br Med J* 1983; **287**:1665–1667.

Lindman RD, Tobin J, Shock NW. Longitudinal studies on the rate of decline in renal function with age. *J Am Geriatr Soc* 1985; **33**: 278–285.

Phillips TL, Rolls BJ, Ledingham JGG, *et al.* Reduced thirst after water deprivation in healthy elderly men. *N Eng J Med* 1984; **311**:753–759.

6 AGEING BONE, MUSCLES AND JOINTS

- The endosteal envelope phenomenon
- Bone collagen
- Osteoporosis
- Vitamin D
- Osteomalacia
- Muscles and joints
- Thresholds for independent life

Bone comes in two forms, cortical and trabecular (or cancellous). Cortical bone forms the dense outer shell of the long bones and the trabecular type bone is the network of thin sheets of bone between the cortical shell.

Bone is composed of living cells and a bone matrix, principally collagen, upon which bone salts are deposited. Throughout life, even after cessation of longitudinal growth, cancellous and cortical bone are constantly being replaced. Changes in the balance between formation and resorption underlie disease affecting the adult skeleton. In both sexes the amount of bone in the body increases until the fourth decade, and then declines. The quantity of bone present at maturity depends upon sex, race, height, body build, posture, exercise and the supply of calcium, protein and vitamin D during growth and development.

THE ENDOSTEAL ENVELOPE PHENOMENON

Bony material lies outside the bone cells and remodelling takes place from the surfaces upon which the cells active in remodelling reside. Three surfaces or envelopes have been defined: the *periosteal* which lines the outside of all bones, the *endosteal* which lines the marrow cavities and covers the trabeculae of cancellous bone, and the *intracortical* or Haversian which lines the Haversian canals. In the normal adult, most bones are inactive.

Remodelling is a local phenomenon and proceeds in a uniform sequence (see Fig. 6.1). First, a localized area of the mesenchyme is activated and osteoclasts are formed which resorb or remove the adjacent bone surface. After about a month the osteoclasts disappear

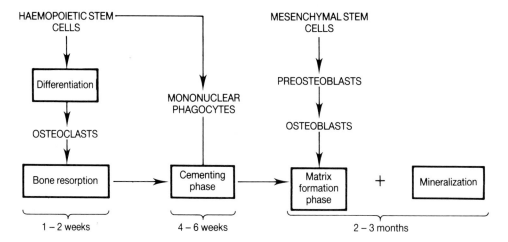

Figure 6.1 Bone remodelling

and are replaced by osteoblasts formed from mesenchymal precursors. Osteoblasts deposit new bone on the previously resorbed surface until finally a resting stage is established. Remodelling units are activated by parathormone (PTH). The time required to complete the sequence is estimated to be from 3 to 4 months.

The periosteal surface is predominantly a bone-forming surface, so the external diameters of bones increase with age. The endosteal surface is predominantly a resorbing surface so the marrow cavity also enlarges with age.

BONE COLLAGEN

The function of collagen is mainly mechanical. Throughout the body collagen fibres are stabilized by a system of covalent interchain cross-links. Both intramolecular and intermolecular cross-links increase with age. The proportion of soluble collagen in human bone and dihydroxylysinonorleucine (DiOH-LNL) both decrease markedly with age. It is not known whether the increasing cross-linkages which strengthen the bone are eventually deleterious, nor whether the change in solubility of collagen affects bone loss. Changes in the cross-linkages are responsible for the type of fractures: few cross-linkages are associated with greenstick fractures seen in children.

OSTEOPOROSIS

There may be two groups of old people with the clinical syndrome of osteoporosis — too little bone of normal composition.

First there are those who, having a small bone mass in adult life, have gradually lost sufficient with advancing years to develop clinical osteoporosis. The second group are those with a precipitating cause such as hyperthyroidism, neoplastic disease, scurvy, malabsorption (e.g. following partial gastrectomy), or spontaneous or iatrogenic Cushing syndrome.

Approximately 90 per cent of bone is fibrous collagen protein, the remainder being mainly calcium and phosphorus. A loss of 30–50 per cent of bone must occur (by excessive resorption over formation) in order to produce osteoporosis. This means an average loss in the skeleton of 50 mg of calcium per day for 20–30 years. No significant changes occur in bone composition with increasing age.

Prolonged immobilization can cause bone loss at any age. Significant bone loss has been demonstrated in a hemiplegic limb as soon as nine weeks after the onset of disability, but this is not found in the presence of passive motion of the limb.

Osteoporosis classically presents at the time of a fracture, either of a vertebral body or of a long bone. A collapse fracture of a vertebral body may present with sudden onset of knife-like back pain, often encircling the girdle. The pain itself is self-limiting and usually lasts about six weeks. Assessment of osteoporosis in the vertebral column is difficult. Radiographs of the spine can be misleading, but points to look for are anterior wedging of the vertebrae and accentuation of the vertical trabeculation of the vertebral body. There is a close correlation between osteoporosis and backache but not between backache and radiographic findings. Chronic bone pain almost certainly indicates some other disorder.

Mobilization remains the mainstay of treatment and prevention. The effects of immobilization and the benefit of exercise were dramatically demonstrated in astronauts. In the early flights significant loss of calcium from bone was demonstrated during a four-day flight. The bone loss was regained by 47 days after the flight, and institution of an exercise programme for later flights prevented such loss. Precipitating causes must be identified and if possible treated. More aggressive approaches include the use of hormone replacement therapy, cyclical biphosphonates, calcium and human growth hormone as well as preventative programmes of exercise.

VITAMIN D

Vitamin D is the name given to a group of fat-soluble secosteroids which act by attaching themselves to macromolecules, thus altering their structure. Vitamin D is found in fish oils, margarine, and in small amounts in eggs and milk. Dietary vitamin D is absorbed from the small intestine, mostly in the form of vitamin D_2 in the presence of bile salts which are needed for the formation of micelles. There is an enterohepatic circulation, vitamin D being secreted in the bile as glucuronides and reabsorbed through the intestinal mucosa. The main source of vitamin D is the conversion in the skin of 7-dehydrocholesterol into vitamin D_3 by the action of ultraviolet light. Some authorities consider that only at times of lack of exposure to sunlight is dietary vitamin D_2 required.

25-hydroxylation occurs on the endoplasmic reticulum of the liver cells, converting vitamin D_3 to 25-hydroxycholecalciferol (25-OH-D3) under the influence of the enzyme vitamin D_3 25-hydroxylase. 25-hydroxy vitamin D_3 then undergoes 1-hydroxylation in the mitochondria of the renal tubular cells. The compound thus formed is 1,25-dihydroxycholecalciferol (1,25-OH$_2$-D3). 1,25-dihydroxy vitamin D_3 increases intestinal absorption of calcium and acts at the renal tubular level to produce reabsorption of calcium from the tubular lumen.

Hypocalcaemia is recognized by the parathyroid glands which in response secrete parathormone. In the kidney, parathormone facilitates the reabsorption of calcium and stimulates the release of 1,25-dihydroxy D_3 which acts alone to increase calcium absorption from the small intestine and together with parathormone to mobilize calcium from bone, thus causing a rise in serum calcium. When serum calcium has reached its normal level the stimulus to parathormone secretion is cut off and the process is stopped.

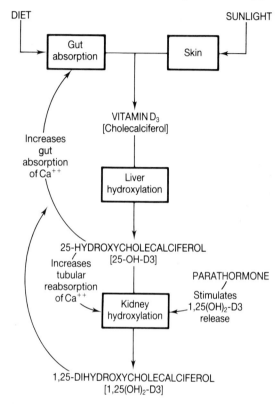

Figure 6.2 Vitamin D metabolism and actions

In hypercalcaemia, the processes are reversed. Calcitonin is secreted from parafollicular C cells in the thyroid gland in response to a raised serum calcium and restores the level to normal. Calcitonin produces its effect by an action on the bone cells, osteoclasts, osteocytes and osteoblasts.

These actions of vitamin D are shown diagrammatically in Fig. 6.2.

OSTEOMALACIA

Lack of vitamin D in elderly people is responsible for the clinical syndrome of osteomalacia. Symptoms include recurrent fractures, difficulty in walking (especially climbing stairs) and a constant low back pain.

Signs are generalized bone tenderness and a waddling gait, associated with proximal myopathy.

Figure 6.3 Looser's zone in right pubic ramus arising from osteomalacia

The presence of Looser's zones (pseudo-fractures) on x-ray over the lateral border of the scapula, first rib, greater trochanter or pubic rami are pathognomonic (see Fig. 6.3). Serum biochemistry may be normal or show a low or normal calcium, a low phosphate and raised alkaline phosphatase. Iliac crest bone biopsy demonstrates widening of the osteoid seams.

The incidence has been put as high as 4 per cent of admissions to geriatric units. Some evidence of osteomalacia has been found in 20 – 30 per cent of women and in about 40 per cent of men with fractures of the proximal femur. Elderly people tend to expose only their hands and faces to sunlight, and the presence of cataracts may necessitate the wearing of a wide-brimmed hat to reduce light exposure to the face (see Chapter 3). Atmospheric pollution also cuts down ultraviolet irradiation. The housebound elderly are particularly at risk since window glass absorbs ultraviolet waves. A vicious circle is set up with lack of exposure to the sun causing deficient vitamin D production, development of back pain and the myopathic gait which makes getting out of chairs and climbing stairs increasingly difficult. Osteomalacia should be suspected in all housebound people.

Elderly people have reduced vitamin D intake. In addition, vitamin D is fat-soluble and needs bile salts for its absorption. Chronic liver disease can lead to bone disease because of a defect in 25 hydroxylation or interference with the entero-hepatic circulation. *Any* cause of malabsorption in the elderly may lead to the development of osteomalacia because of the enterohepatic circulation of vitamin D and its fat-solubility.

The renal tubule is the site of the 1-hydroxylation, and this is the explanation for the early occurrence of bone disease in disorders affecting the renal tubule rather than the glomerulus. It has been suggested that mitochondrial enzyme induction in the liver might be the reason why epileptic patients on therapy with anticonvulsant drugs develop osteomalacia, cholecalciferol being metabolized to inactive metabolites. Patients with epilepsy who remain on anticonvulsant treatment despite symptoms of osteomalacia have been treated with vitamin D in doses of 4000 units per day.

Prevention and treatment. Exposure to ultraviolet light encourages vitamin D formation. Supplementation of dietary intake by switching from butter to margarine which is fortified is sensible. Treatment with vitamin D is necessary in the frank case of osteomalacia, and in people with neither renal impairment nor malabsorption there are no benefits in using the expensive 'one-alpha' preparation. Prolonged daily usage or too high a dose can lead to hypercalcaemia. Bone pain and tenderness may become worse about two days after starting treatment but tend to improve after one week. Maintenance therapy should be titrated according to the clinical response to treatment.

MUSCLES AND JOINTS

Muscle strength declines with age, from its peak values in the early 20s to 40s. Muscle strength in some muscles may decline by as much as 5 – 7 per cent a year from the age of 70. These declines are associated with parallel reductions in muscle mass. There are changes in both the numbers and size of muscle fibres, affecting predominantly type II fibres. These changes are probably due to reductions in the numbers of anterior horn cells in the spinal cord that innervate skeletal muscles, leading to progressive loss of muscle mass and weakness.

Such reductions in muscle strength are paralleled by similar changes in physical capacity, including maximal oxygen consumption, airways resistance, and joint flexibility. Reduced range of movement across a joint may also lead to further wasting and weakness, as will any damage within a joint.

Osteoarthrosis is so common with increasing age (up to 85 per cent at ages 75–79) that it is tempting to assume that it is part of 'normal' ageing. However, the changes that occur in the cartilage of osteoarthritic joints are not the same as those that occur in old joints. Cartilage consists of chondrocytes, collagen, proteoglycans (chondroitan sulphate and keratin sulphate) and water. Adult cartilage contains less water, and its proteoglycan structure and content changes, although the total level remains the same. The number of chondrocytes also falls.

By contrast, in osteoarthrosis the water content of cartilage is higher because the collagen becomes disrupted, and less densely woven together, and drinks in water like a sponge. As the cartilage becomes more damaged, chondrocytes start to divide and become much more active, producing a wide range of destructive enzymes (including collagenase) as well as attempting to repair damage by production of more collagen, proteoglycans and hyaluronic acid. Microfractures occur in the bone around the joint and lead to cysts and sclerosis. Erosions in the cartilage are associated with proliferation of bone and osteophyte formation at the joint margins. The underlying aetiological factors are not known, although genetic factors, occupation and/or trauma are probably implicated.

THRESHOLDS FOR INDEPENDENT LIFE

Age-related declines in physical capacity are of no significance in themselves until they prevent a person from carrying out necessary tasks (see Fig. 6.4). Many elderly people find it almost impossible to get out of a low chair which has no arms. This is because their muscles cannot generate sufficient force to overcome their body weight. An acute illness or a spell of bed-rest may accelerate the loss of strength, and this explains why an apparently mild illness can have a devastating effect on a person who is on the threshold of being unable to carry out activities of daily living. Much of the rehabilitation required by elderly people during and after acute illnesses is essentially aimed at improving muscle strength, flexibility and stamina. Even in old age improvements in muscle strength and joint flexibility can be achieved of similar scale to those experienced by younger people. For example, regular use of the legs to lift weights by people in their

80s and 90s can lead to about 15 per cent improvement in muscle strength. More importantly it enables some chair-fast subjects to get up without help. Regular exercise can therefore help overcome some

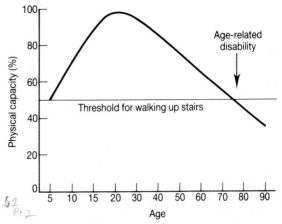

Figure 6.4 Age-related changes in muscle strength: a threshold for independent life

of the age associated changes, and raises the question of whether such changes are truly due to ageing, or more correctly attributed to lack of activity.

Key points

- Bone collagen cross-linkages increase with age. The significance of these changes in determining bone strength is not known. Greenstick fractures are common in young children who have few cross-linkages.
- Osteoporosis is defined as too little bone of normal composition. Bone mass reaches a peak in early adult life and then falls, rapidly after the female menopause.
- Osteomalacia is due to vitamin D deficiency, which is often the result of poor dietary intake and/or inadequate sunlight exposure. Malabsorption, chronic liver disease and chronic renal failure are rarer causes.
- Muscle strength reaches a peak during the young adult years and then declines, probably because of reductions in the numbers of anterior horn cells in the spinal cord.
- Osteoarthrosis is *not* due to ageing changes in joints. It is associated with thinning of articular cartilage, whereas cartilage tends to increase in thickness with age.

- Physical exercise may ameliorate some of the adverse changes in muscle strength and joint flexibility.

FURTHER READING

Aniansson A, Grimby G, Rungren A, Svanborg A, Olander J. Physical training in old men. *Age and Ageing* 1980;9:186–187.

Fentem PH, Bassey EJ, Turnbull, NB. *The New Case for Exercise.* Health Education Authority, 1988.

Kay MMB, Galpin J, Makinodan T (eds). *Aging, Immunity and Arthritic Disease.* Raven Press, New York, 1980.

Shepherd R. *Physical Activity and Ageing,* 2nd edn. Croom Helm, London, 1987.

Smith EL, Serfass RC (eds). *Exercise and Aging: The Scientific Basis.* Enslow Publishers, Hillside, NJ, 1981.

Smith R. Osteoporosis: causes and management. *Br Med J* 1987; **294**:329–332.

Young A. Exercise physiology in geriatric practice. *Acta Med Scand* (suppl) 1986; **711**:227–232.

7 THE AGEING BRAIN

- Brain structure
- Brain functional areas
- Forgetfulness and intelligence
- Dementia
- Other ageing changes

The brains of humans have developed to a remarkable extent, giving us huge cerebral hemispheres that sit on top of the more primitive mid and hind brain stuctures that control basic life processes.

BRAIN STRUCTURE

During embryonic development the brain surface is smooth up to four months. It then becomes irregular, producing the characteristic ridges and troughs — gyri and sulci — of the brain surface. These undulations increase the surface area to around 30 times that of the skull size, thus packing in much more grey matter. The grey matter is made up of nerve cells and the white matter is made up of nerve fibres streaming from the cells. Each nerve cell has a fibre (axon) transmitting impulses away from the cell, and many more connections (dendrites) connecting the brain cell with other cells.

With age the brain volume becomes smaller by about 10 per cent of the young adult volume. The gyri become more prominent and the sulci deeper, and the ventricles enlarge. It is likely that old brains contain fewer nerve cells, although since there are many millions of brain cells no-one has ever counted them to prove whether this really is so. The difficulty of studying true ageing changes, rather than the effects of pathological processes, must be borne in mind. In dementia syndromes, dramatic loss of neurones is typical and it is impossible to be sure that human brains studied after death were not affected by early stages of a dementia syndrome.

It appears that cells are lost at different rates in different parts of the brain. Neuronal loss in the cortex is estimated to be about 1 per cent per year, but much faster rates of loss occur in the basal ganglia and cerebellum. The locus coeruleus, which has a large number of catecholaminergic cells, loses cells at the rate of about 40 per cent per year after the age of 60. Animal studies have demonstrated very little change in the numbers of neurones and an increase in glial cells.

The number of dendrites decreases with age, which may be due to a reduction in the rate at which they are renewed, or may be a genuine loss. The loss of dendrites is associated with a reduction in synaptic activity, and presumably communication and information processing is reduced. The changes seen in Alzheimer's disease are severe, but the significance of the much milder changes in normal aged brains is not known.

BRAIN FUNCTIONAL AREAS

Areas of the brain perform specific functions (see Fig. 7.1). In the motor area of the cortex the body is represented from the foot at the midline to the hand at the lateral edge. A comparable sensory area of the cortex receives information from the body. These motor and sensory areas are interconnected with other parts of the brain through the branching network of dendrites. This permits the fine control of movement, and the coordination between eye and hand.

The frontal lobes of the brain are large and were formerly considered to be 'silent'. Large amounts of frontal cortex can be destroyed and the person can live on quite normally. However, the frontal lobe has an important role in the control of behaviour, attention and emotion. Damage to the frontal lobes can give rise to a characteristic syndrome of disinhibited, crude behaviour. Surgical damage (prefrontal leucotomy) is still used as a treatment for severe, and otherwise untreatable, depression.

The temporal lobes and adjacent deep stuctures (hippocampus, nucleus of Meynert, etc.) are concerned with memory. Study of the pathology of Alzheimer's disease has shown that it appears to strike these areas most severely. Ideas about the structure of memory are expanding rapidly. Short-term memory is probably stored in the form of electrical potential differences between neurones for a matter of a few minutes. These electrical changes then lead to the

Figure 7.1 Lobes of the brain and their functions

The pathways that the axons follow from cortical neurones cross over in the brainstem. As a result, the left motor cortex controls movement of the right side of the body and vice versa.

The parietal lobe is located between the back of the brain (the occipital cortex where vision resides) and the sensory cortex. It is concerned with recognition of objects and spatial awareness. Damage to this part of the brain was the cause of the symptoms that gave the title to Oliver Sacks' celebrated book (and opera) *The Man who Mistook his Wife for a Hat.*

laying down of memory by protein synthesis for a period of a few hours. Finally, long-term memory is held by changes in the dendrites and their interconnections.

Acute losses of memory — amnestic syndromes — are associated with damage to the hippocampus, thalamus and limbic system. No impairment of thinking, personality, attention or concentration occurs, and it is usual for very remote memory to be unaffected, suggesting that this sort of memory is laid down very widely.

Dominance. Right- and left-handedness are indicators of which side of the brain is dominant. In right-handers, the left side is dominant, but a proportion of left-handers also have left-sided brain dominance. Speech is a complex function, and the speech areas are located in the dominant hemisphere in the frontal, temporal and parietal regions. Interestingly, while speech may be lost if the left side of the brain is damaged by a stroke, the ability to sing may not be affected. Second languages may also be unimpaired.

The mid brain and hind brain. These parts of the brain are concerned with basic life-supporting functions (breathing, arousal, maintenance of circulation) and with control of posture and movement. They are also extensively connected with cortical areas.

FORGETFULNESS AND INTELLIGENCE

Forgetting things is a normal everyday behaviour. A young child forgetting to take an exercise book to school is considered quite normal, whereas an elderly person forgetting to take money on a shopping trip may think this indicates early dementia. It is often necessary to reassure elderly people that such forgetfulness is normal, and the term 'benign senile forgetfulness' has been coined for this problem.

Both young and old forget things at similar rates, but in older people the ability to remember strings of numbers or items on a list is less. This may be due to true ageing changes, but more probably reflects a cohort effect. People born in 1900 had less schooling or exposure to various media, and less need to remember strings of numbers for the telephone. Their performance on such 'intelligence' tests is therefore less good than by people born a generation later. In fact there is good evidence from longitudinal studies that many aspects of intelligence do not deteriorate with increasing age. Speed of response, which is a factor in some intelligence tests, also declines with age and may make elderly people appear to do less well in tests. Some of the tests themselves are rather childish and may irritate elderly subjects, thus leading to poor motivation and performance.

DEMENTIA

For normal brain functioning, adequate supplies of energy, oxygen, vitamins and hormones are required. Interference with these basic needs will lead to global functional deterioration (i.e. confusion) which, provided the interference is only temporary, can recover. By contrast, the damage caused by dementing diseases is permanent and progressive.

The typical findings in Alzheimer's dementia are of diffuse cortical atrophy, with loss of neurones. Neurofibrillary tangles and vacuoles (holes) are found inside the neurones, together with plaques of amyloid deposits. These changes are most marked in the hippocampus, the temporal–parietal–occipital junction, and in the nucleus basalis of Meynert. In addition to these changes, the interconnections between neurones wither away. Alzheimer's disease also leads to reductions in neurotransmitters, particularly acetylcholine, and corresponding reductions in enzymes such as choline acetyl transferase. Attempts simply to substitute the deficient neurotransmitter (in the same way as L-dopa is used to substitute for low levels of dopamine in Parkinson's disease) have not proved successful, demonstrating that the fundamental nature of the disease is not fully understood (see Table 7.1).

Table 7.1 Pathological changes in Alzheimer's disease

Senile plaques: granular fragments surrounded by astrocytes, often containing microglia, and amyloid

Neurofibrillary tangles: thickened neurofibrils which swing around the cell nucleus and form a circular shape in the cytoplasm

Granulo-vacuolar degeneration: affected neurones show clusters of intracytoplasmic vacuoles each of which shows a dense round central granule

The brains of normal old people are not immune from similar changes: plaques of amyloid deposition, intraneuronal tangles and vacuoles all occur. The difference is in their numbers and distribution. It is generally accepted that dementia is due to structural and irreversible damage to the brain, rather than an acceleration of a normal ageing process.

Alzheimer's disease can run in families. When it does, around 50 per cent of all children are affected, suggesting an autosomal dominant mode of inheritance. The gene for familial Alzheimer's disease is on chromosome 21, and this discovery led to further excitement because Down's syndrome (trisomy 21) is associated with a dementia, and very similar pathological changes in the brain. The trail went very cold when it was found that the gene responsible was not the same in different families with Alzheimer's disease, nor was the gene implicated in the much more common non-familial disease.

OTHER AGEING CHANGES

In addition to the cortical changes, the peripheral nervous system declines with age. Awareness of pain, touch, temperature, joint position and vibration sense all get worse with age. Indeed it is quite normal for vibration sense to be absent at the ankles in elderly people. Some of these changes may be due to reductions in nerve conduction velocity.

The control of posture and balance also decline, making old people more prone to falls, and to adopt a broader-based walking pattern. It is unusual to see a very old person who does not walk with a gait reminiscent of early Parkinsonism. The mechanisms for changes in gait, posture and balance are not understood. It is likely that many different but interrelated mechanisms are involved. These may include neuronal loss in the basal ganglia and cortex, reduction in reaction times, muscle atrophy, changes in labyrinthine and visual perception, and reductions in proprioception.

Key points

- Brain weight, volume, cell numbers, and dendrites decline with age, although there are marked regional variations within the brain.
- Brain functions are localized. Apart from the motor cortex and sensory cortex, the parietal lobe is concerned with recognition, the frontal lobes with control of behaviour, attention and emotion, and the temporal lobes, hippocampus and nucleus of Meynert with memory. Speech is complex with multiple association areas in the temporal, parietal and frontal regions.
- Not all forgetfulness heralds the onset of dementia. Old and young people suffer with forgetfulness to a similar extent.
- Alzheimer's disease is characterized by senile plaques, neurofibrillary tangles and granulo-vacuolar degeneration. Normal old brains show the same kind of changes, but in Alzheimer's disease the amount of change is far greater and the distribution of changes is most marked in the hippocampus, the temporal–parietal–occipital junction, and in the nucleus basalis of Meynert.
- The characteristic neurotransmitter deficit in Alzheimer's disease is of acetylcholine with reductions in the enzyme choline acetyl transferase.

FURTHER READING

Brayne C, Calloway P. Normal ageing, impaired cognitive function, and senile dementia of the Alzheimer's type: a continuum? *Lancet*, 1988; **i**:1265–1267.

Jarvik LF. Thoughts on the psychology of ageing. *Am Psychol* 1975; May: 576–583.

Jorm AF. *The Epidemiology of Alzheimer's Disease and Related Disorders.* Chapman & Hall, London, 1990.

Prusiner SB. Some speculations about prions, amyloid and Alzheimer's disease. *N Eng J Med* 1984; **310**:661–663.

Rinn WE. Mental decline in normal ageing: a review. *J Geriatr Psychiat Neurol* 1988; **1**:144–158.

Tanzi RE, Gusella JF, Watkins PC, *et al.* Amyloid B protein gene: cDNA, mRNA distribution, and genetic linkage near the Alzheimer locus. *Science* 1987; **235**:880–884.

8 THE AGEING CARDIOVASCULAR SYSTEM

- Structural changes
- Heart rate
- Blood pressure
- Other points

Changes in the cardiovascular system have long been thought of as the basis for the general physiological decline attributed to ageing. Leonardo da Vinci wrote that the cause of ageing was 'veins which by the thickening of their tunics in the old, restricts the passage of their blood and by this lack of nourishment destroys the life of the aged without any fever, the old coming to fail little by little in slow death'. The cardiovascular system exemplifies the dilemma of physiology versus pathology in the normal ageing process. It is now evident that the physiological changes associated with age are comparatively minor and amount to slightly poorer function whereas the pathological changes (especially those of atherosclerotic coronary artery disease) are severe, extremely damaging, and often life-threatening.

STRUCTURAL CHANGES

Cardiovascular structural changes with age are well documented. Aortic elasticity declines (this is due to changes in the media, not the intimal changes of atherosclerosis) and the aorta commonly widens (seen clinically on chest x-rays as a widened aortic arch). The elasticity changes mean that systolic blood pressure may thus rise slightly with age. Heart valves (especially the aortic) can become less mobile in a proportion of elderly people (exacerbated by atheromatous disease and calcification) and cause the commonly heard ejection systolic murmur. Degeneration and calcification of the mitral valve can result in either apical ejection murmurs or the more common pansystolic mitral incompetence/regurgitant murmur. Age changes in the myocardium result in the accumulation of the 'waste product' lipofuscin and the so-called 'brown atrophy'.

HEART RATE

The effect of age on the resting heart rate is equivocal but it appears that the heart rate increase in response to stress is probably less effective in advanced old age. Cardiac output falls slightly with advancing age (about 1 per cent a year) and this, together with the slight rise in systolic blood pressure means that the systemic peripheral resistance is somewhat increased. The changes in cardiac output are probably related to the small decreases in body size that occur, and to the fact that slightly less blood is pumped per heart beat per unit body size.

There is a decrease in the number of conducting cells in the SA node with age and some increase in fibrous tissue, but very little effect on the AV node. Atrial fibrillation is more common in the elderly but is more often due to atherosclerosis than to fibrosis.

BLOOD PRESSURE

Systolic and diastolic blood pressures rise with age in most Western populations, but as this is not universal it is unlikely to be a true ageing process — Strehler's theory — neither is it always progressive or irreversible. Even though vascular ageing changes may occur that predispose to hypertension, other compensating factors may be important (diet, physical fitness, etc.).

Hypertension in the elderly, its definition and its possible treatment are still highly contentious. Blood pressure needs to be measured accurately and over a period of time. Blood pressure can be labile and readings can change with posture; hence lying and standing measurements should be made.

Although 'hypertension' must be seen in the context of the individual, it may be thought that biological rather than chronological age is a better guide to possible intervention measures. Evidence from clinical trials suggests that treatment is beneficial up to the age of 80 years, and for levels above 160/100 (phase V). The end-organ effects of sustained hypertension (angina, left ventricular failure, etc.) may obviously influence the management. If hypertension is found to be part of a generalized atheromatous state, thought should be given to the issue of whether in that particular person the physiological parameters have been set at a new 'higher' level determined by the disease process and are necessary for function. Changing this may cause more not less damage being inflicted. The side effects of drug management in the very old must be weighed against the expected benefits (morbidity and mortality reduction) and be carefully examined.

Hypotension is a common finding in elderly people, especially that which is posturally related. This usually results either from the use of drugs with a hypotensive effect (e.g. diuretics, major tranquillizers, L-dopa, alcohol, etc.), or more rarely, from impairment in the baroreceptor reflex mechanism (diabetic neuropathy, tabes dorsalis, Parkinson's disease, Shy–Drager syndrome, etc.).

Cardiac hypertrophy. Cardiovascular disease is a very common finding in an ageing population (depending on the definition of cardiovascular disease and the completeness of the physical and laboratory investigations). A large sub-population of the elderly have enlarged hearts but as hypertrophy (increase in size due to increased work load over long periods) is not inevitable in all elderly individuals it cannot be considered an ageing process.

Peripheral resistance. Organ perfusion decreases with age, as indicated by data from peripheral resistance to blood flow and clearance of certain substances. These changes in organ perfusion may be secondary to either less blood being supplied to the capillaries due to atheroma of the large vessels or reductions in cardiac output (not a major influence). Organ perfusion can also be altered secondary to changes in tissue (metabolic demands or loss of compliance). Peripheral resistance increases with age and this probably plays a role in decreasing blood flow.

OTHER POINTS

The efficiency of the oxygen transport system declines with age. So, to a small extent, does thermoregulation, which in part depends on heat conduction by cutaneous blood flow which becomes more sluggish. A change in one part of the cardiovascular system influences every other and it is difficult to distinguish primary from secondary age changes. However, most of the changes with age are probably due to a small number of factors which are intrinsic.

Normal cardiovascular ageing may be hard to find in Western societies, but we must not let the common pathological changes found in elderly patients influence the fact that normal ageing means slight and sometimes subtle changes in measurements. Clinical findings may include a slight rise in blood pressure and possibly atrial fibrillation and ejection systolic 'flow' murmurs.

KEY POINTS

- Cardiovascular physiological changes with age are minor, pathological changes severe.
- Structural changes often include a widening aortic arch and ejection systolic murmurs.

- The heart rate increase in response to stress is less effective.
- Cardiac output falls slightly with advancing age (about 1 per cent a year).
- Atrial fibrillation is common but is more often due to atherosclerosis than to fibrosis.
- Systolic and diastolic blood pressure rise with age in Western populations (though it is not universal).
- Blood pressure needs to be measured accurately and over a period of time.
- Treatment of hypertension in the elderly needs to take into account 'biological' age, end-organ damage and potential side-effects.
- Postural hypotension is a common finding in elderly people.

FURTHER READING

Finch CE, Schneider EL (eds). *Handbook of the Biology of Ageing*. Van Nostrand Reinhold, New York, 1985.

9 THE AGEING RESPIRATORY SYSTEM

- Structural changes
- Functional changes
- Examining the elderly chest
- Chest x-ray

The respiratory system comprises airways that transport inspired air to the alveoli where transfer of gases takes place, and the supporting structures of the chest wall. All of these are affected by ageing, and many of the age changes are accelerated by smoking.

The large airways are kept open by rings of cartilage. As the airways branch out and narrow the support that keeps them open is provided by the elastic recoil of the lung parenchymal tissue, and cartilage is not present in these very small diameter airways.

STRUCTURAL CHANGES

With ageing, the elasticity of the lungs declines. This leads to early closure of the very small airways on breathing out, with trapping of air. The reduction in parenchymal support to the airways tends to reduce their overall size and makes the lung more compliant — or distensible.

These two trends of loss of elasticity and increased distensibility make the lungs occupy a bigger space. On chest x-rays it may look as if the lungs are over-inflated. The diaphragm is flat and the ribs become more horizontal. The x-ray appearances are similar to those seen in emphysema; indeed the loss of elasticity and the air-trapping lead to a progressive dilatation of the alveoli and a form of emphysema, very similar to that seen in patients with alpha-1 antitrypsin deficiency, in which the lung parenchyma is 'digested' away. In smokers, these changes are aggravated and are associated with mucous cell hypertrophy and inflammatory changes as well.

Table 9.1 Changes in the chest wall and lungs

Chest wall
Stiff costovertebral and costochondral joints
Increased AP diameter due to kyphosis
Wasting of respiratory muscles
Increased use of diaphragm

Lung
Alveoli support diminished
Increased mucous glands
Reduced elasticity
Increased physiological dead space
Reduced surface area for gas exchange
Reduced capillary circulation

In addition to the ageing changes within the lung, the chest wall ages. Perhaps the most dramatic is the kyphosis that is common in many elderly people. This is due to degeneration in intervertebral discs and may be aggravated by osteoporosis with thoracic vertebral collapse. Kyphosis reduces the diameter of the chest, and with calcification of costal cartilages, makes the chest wall more rigid. The respiratory muscles, along with other skeletal muscle, also become weaker with age. These changes are brought together in Table 9.1.

FUNCTIONAL CHANGES

The ageing changes in structure lead to predictable functional effects. The volume of air that can be expired in one second (FEV_1) falls because of the reduction in elasticity and air-trapping, and because of weakness of respiratory muscles. The decline in FEV_1, peak flow rate, and forced vital capacity can be predicted from standard equations. It is necessary to take into account sex, height and smoking habit, all of which will affect lung ventilation.

The relative proportions of lung volumes change with age (see Fig. 9.1). The tidal volume remains about the same at about half a litre, but the inspiratory reserve and expiratory reserve volumes both decline and the residual volume increases quite markedly.

that the elderly person has lower than expected lung function.

Cross-sectional studies also tend to over-estimate the loss of lung function with age. The longitudinal rates of decline found are smaller than those obtained from cross-sectional studies. This may be due to a form of selection bias. To remain in a longitudinal study, a subject must survive, and survival is associated with better lung function.

Gas exchange is also affected by ageing. Ventilation of the lung is matched by blood flow. Areas of the lung with less ventilation automatically receive less blood, and vice versa. When a person is sitting upright, the ventilation to the lung bases is higher than to the upper parts of the lung. This is matched by increased blood flow to the bases. The tendency to early closure of airways, with air trapping, reduces the ventilation of the bases, and leads to a mismatch between ventilation and perfusion. The result of this is an age-related reduction in the arterial oxygen saturation.

On exertion, the respiratory system is stressed and the functional reserve capacity has to be used. With age, the reserve capacity is much more limited. In particular, the weakness of respiratory muscles contributes to the exertional breathlessness seen in elderly people. It is likely that training can improve

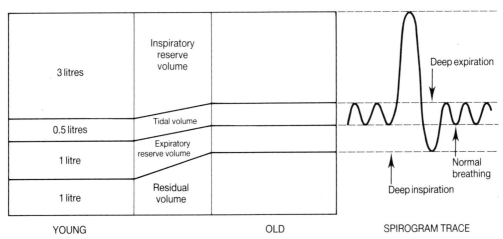

Figure 9.1 Lung volumes of young and old people

Although data from cross-sectional studies show an apparently linear decline, small studies of very elderly people suggest that the rate of decline increases in the very old. If data from younger subjects are extrapolated to the very old, this will lead to predicted values being too high, and the assumption

respiratory efficiency, even in the very old, and thus reduce some of the adverse consquences of ageing on the respiratory system.

It is often forgotten that the lung is also an immunological organ coping with the challenges of many different potential allergens and pathogens with each lung full of air. With age, the lung defence mechanisms (mucous production, local antibodies, cell mediated immunity) wane, making elderly people much more susceptible to infection.

EXAMINING THE ELDERLY CHEST

Examination of the chest comprises a ritual of assessing the chest wall, checking whether the trachea is central, gauging expansion by eye and hand (but seldom tape-measure), followed by percussion, tactile and vocal fremitus, and listening for abnormal sounds. Much of this has been demonstrated to be of virtually no value at all, with very poor agreement between doctors on the presence or absence of signs, and low validity when compared with the 'gold standards' of chest x-ray and CT scanning. However, some parts of the examination are worth carrying out.

Respiratory rate

Counting the respiratory rate is one of the most useful screening examinations for elderly people. At rest the normal respiratory rate will be around 15 breaths per minute. The anxiety of a clinical examination may push this up to 20 per minute. With respiratory distress caused by heart failure, pneumonia, pulmonary embolus, asthma, etc., one of the first mechanisms to maintain gas transfer and avoid hypoxia is to increase respiratory rate. It is not until rates increase to 35–40 per minute that a person looks obviously short of breath, so it is necessary to count the rate over at least half a minute to pick up less severe problems.

Chest movement

In normal elderly people the chest wall does not move as much as in young people. It may be difficult to decide if expansion is symmetrical because the chest wall moves so little. Abdominal respiration is not affected, and it is obvious that anything that limits abdominal respiration (e.g. abdominal surgery, abdominal pain, tight corsets, gross obesity) will have a disproportionate effect on respiratory efficiency, and lead to hypoxia.

Breath sounds

Doctors are taught to listen for crackles in the lung

bases as a sign of heart failure. These crackles are probably caused by the opening and closing of very small airways. In elderly people, the increased fine crackles of heart failure are masked by much coarser noises produced by the air-trapping caused by loss of lung elasticity. Such noises should not be assummed to be pathological.

CHEST X-RAY

In a sick elderly person a chest x-ray is an essential investigation, regardless of the presence or absence of signs or symptoms. The elderly person's chest x-ray may tell a story, and the best way to understand the story is to make the effort of getting hold of old films which may help in interpretation.

Common changes are calcification from old tuberculosis, calcification in chondral cartilages, pleural calcification from past pneumonia, old rib fractures, and more rarely occupational dust exposures.

A major problem for elderly people is to adopt the required posture for a good quality PA erect chest x-ray. All too often a supine film is done, usually not in full inspiration, and with a degree of rotation. This makes it impossible to determine whether effusions are present, makes heart size and the mediastinum impossible to assess. Sick elderly people are not easy to x-ray well, and a sympathetic and experienced radiographer is essential.

KEY POINTS

- The elasticity of the lungs declines with age, leading to early closure of very small airways and air-trapping. Parenchymal support also declines, reducing the size of the lungs and making them more compliant.
- The chest wall becomes more rigid with age (owing to kyphosis and calcification of costal cartilage), increasing the work of respiration.
- The structural changes lead to reductions in FEV_1 and other indicators of lung function. The rate of reduction is markedly affected by smoking.
- Arterial oxygen saturation falls with age because of ventilation–perfusion mismatching occurring at the lung bases.
- Counting the respiratory rate is one of the most useful parts of chest examination. Basal crackles are almost universal in the chests of older smokers.
- Always try to obtain a good quality PA chest x-ray, and any previous old films for comparison.

FURTHER READING

Edge JR, Millard FJC, Reid L, Simon G. The radiographic appearance of the chest in persons of advanced age. *Br J Radiol* 1964; **37**:769–774.

Milne JS. *Clinical Effects of Ageing: A Longitudinal Study.* Croom Helm, London, 1985.

Mittman C, Edelman NH, Norris AH, Shock NW. Relationship between chest wall and pulmonary compliance and age. *J Appl Physiol* 1965; **20**:1211-1216.

Spiteri MA, Cook DG, Clarke SW. Reliability of eliciting physical signs in the examination of the chest. *Lancet* 1988; **i**:873–875.

Thurlbeck WM, Angus GE. Growth and ageing of normal human lung. *Chest* 1975; **67**:3s–7s.

10 THE AGEING ENDOCRINE SYSTEM

- The menopause
- Hormone replacement therapy
- Men
- Sexuality
- Other endocrine organs

The changes that occur in the endocrine system with age were once thought to be the sole cause of the generalized ageing process, and hence that this process could be reversed by the replacement of numerous hormones. 'Ageing' is now seen to be far more complex but replacement of some of the previously thought non-essential hormonal loss is gaining importance.

THE MENOPAUSE

The menopause is defined as the cessation of menstrual periods but is associated with numerous other bodily changes. Menstruation usually becomes irregular before finally stopping, and some women suffer severe physical and mental symptoms associated with the hormonal changes. These include flushing/sweating attacks, altered libido, mucosal changes in the vagina with some dryness and periods of melancholy or even frank depression. During this time the levels of circulating and urinary gonadotrophins — follicle stimulating hormone (FSH) and luteinizing hormone (LH) — are raised, probably reflecting the lowered levels of circulating oestrogens causing a negative feedback on the hypothalamus. With increasing age the oestrogen found in the urine decreases to very low levels. In these elderly women oestrone is the main circulating hormone derived by conversion of plasma androstenedione of adrenal cortical origin, and this conversion increases with age. In addition to the ovaries producing less hormones, the germ cells in the ovary are also affected by age. The quality of the oocytes declines, evidenced by an increase in chromosomal abnormalities in older women, the most notable result being trisomy of chromosome 21 resulting in Down's syndrome. It has been postulated that oocytes that have spent longer in the ovary are more prone to damage by radiation, infection, autoantibody effects, etc. Eventually the postmenopausal ovary fails to respond to the gonadotrophic hormones and it becomes increasingly fibrotic.

For a few years prior to the menopause the uterus increasingly fails to support pregnancy, probably as a result of the physical changes in the uterus and altered hormonal balance//Following the menopause the uterus slowly atrophies/ In postmenopausal women the vagina contracts, shortening the organ and gradually decreasing the size of the lumen. There is loss of elasticity and the epithelium becomes thin, pale and dry./These changes usually occur slowly and imperceptably and should not interfere with sexual intercourse even in the very elderly. However, the hormonal changes that especially affect the epithelium (causing dryness) can be clinically significant, cause discomfort and distress and need to be recognized and treated with local hormone cream or HRT.

/With ageing there is a gradual replacement of glandular breast tissue with fat. Breast carcinoma is the leading malignant cause of death amongst women, and the risk increases with age./Particular attention should be paid to education, self-examining techniques and screening with mammography.

Con.

HORMONE REPLACEMENT THERAPY (HRT)

This initially controversial topic is becoming increasingly important as its protagonists point out its positive effects: the lessening and perhaps avoiding of all the unpleasant side-effects of the menopause, but with the added value of increased psychological well-being (looking and feeling better). In addition there is the protective effect on postmenopausal osteoporosis with its devastating resultant morbidity and mortality from fractures (especially of the neck of femur) in advancing years. New regimens (oestrogen alone, at low dosage or combined with other hormones) are still being developed and evaluated.

The antagonists are concerned about the continued stimulation of organs that biologically and physiologically are naturally failing. There may be an increased risk of uterine/endometrial cancer. As menopausal symptoms are temporary many clinicians agree to short courses of HRT, but extended treatments (favoured by women themselves and backed by some doctors in view of the potential for preventing osteoporosis) are becoming increasingly common. Any effects on the female cardiovascular or other systems have yet to be fully evaluated and many women are precluded because of previous or current disease. Most courses involve time 'off' hormones to allow withdrawal bleeding and to lessen the risk of endometrial carcinoma, yet perpetuating 'menstruation' possibly into old age. Hormonal preparations which give all the protective effects without withdrawal bleeds are being considered.

MEN

The ageing of the male reproductive system is a gradual process. It probably has a variable period of onset. Although devotees of Woody Allen movies would feel there is a lot of evidence for a 'male menopause' or 'andropause', it usually passes without major physical side-effects or psychological trauma. There is no decline in the size or weight of the testes and spermatozoa continue to be produced into old age and are viable. The secretion of testosterone decreases in elderly men. There is fibrous change in the trabeculae of the corpus spongiosum, followed by sclerosis of the arteries and veins. Similar changes occur in the corpora cavernosa.

After the fifth decade the prostate shows less secretory activity and degenerative changes begin which further lessen secretions. Nodular hyperplasia within the stroma of the prostate gland is very common in Caucasians after the age of 50. Carcinoma of the prostate increases in frequency with age and should be carefully looked for in elderly men.

SEXUALITY

Sex drive (libido) is said to decline with age and ejaculation time lengthens. There is, however, considerable variation and numerous other factors have to be taken into account — such as the general health of the person and that of their partner, their sexual needs and wishes viewed over time. The influence of society's views should not be underestimated. Currently sex in old age is seen in some way as being perverse. (Imagine the 'difficulty' if two residents in an old people's home wanted to have sex and needed a degree of privacy and even help to achieve it.) There are no norms for adults: sex should be mutually enjoyable and desired by both partners, at any frequency and at any age. Homosexual relationships are as valid as heterosexual and this aspect of sexuality should not be overlooked or devalued in the elderly.

OTHER ENDOCRINE ORGANS

The endocrine response to stress declines somewhat with age yet there is no evidence to show that this is due to a deficiency in the pituitary–adrenal axis. Underactivity of the adrenals (Addison's disease) does occur in the elderly whereas overactivity (Cushing's disease) is extremely rare over 70.

Insulin deficiency appears to be strongly age-related. In glucose tolerance tests the ability to utilize the glucose load declines with increasing age. The deterioration is so large that many elderly lie in the 'diabetic' category. Whether or not these people are suffering from diabetes mellitus is debatable, although progressively higher blood glucose levels are associated with increased mortality, particularly from heart attacks and strokes. It is not clear whether this change is due to ageing or disease.

The thyroid gland of even very elderly people maintains adequate function. The secretion rate of T4 decreases with age whilst plasma T4 levels do not. The TSH response is unchanged. Thyroid function tests may be altered during illness — the 'sick euthyroid' syndrome with a low T4 but also a low TSH (hypopituitarism being excluded). There are lower levels of plasma T3 circulating in the elderly. It has been postulated that since this is the active hormone there may be a decrease in the effective hormone with ageing. However TSH levels do not rise, so there would also have to be a deficiency in the negative feedback mechanism.

Diagnostic problems are often encountered in thyroid disease. Hypothyroidism (myxoedema) is a condition that can be diagnosed late because the symptoms and signs are subtle (constipation, dry skin and hair, lethargy, puffy features) and of slow onset (deeper voice, tendency to cold intolerance, etc.). The symptoms are also accepted as normal age changes by the patient (and often by the doctor as well); and as constipation, dry skin, tiredness and cold intolerance occur commonly in normal elderly people, a high index of suspicion is necessary. It is said that patients who are seen regularly by carer and doctor are the ones that are missed (the 'classic' case with a pulse of 40 and slow relaxing ankle jerks being a doctor's mother!).

Hyperthyroidism or thyrotoxicosis can also be difficult to diagnose. Patients may present classically, but the 'masked' or 'apathetic' presentation (general debility and inability to cope) with few of the usual symptoms and signs is not uncommon. Thyroid function tests are a useful screening tool in unusual cases of ill-health.

In normal old age the endocrine glands perform their functions and few specific changes are evident (some prostatic enlargement in men, altered breast tissue in women). Other findings often accepted as 'ageing' and hence normal should be viewed as pathological and investigated.

Key points

- The female menopause may be associated with marked physical and mental symptoms.
- Circulating FSH and LH levels are raised via negative feedback of lowered oestrogen levels on the hypothalamus.
- Oestrone is the main circulating hormone.
- Chromosomal abnormalities in the oocytes increases (e.g. trisomy of chromosome 21).
- Clinical symptoms of hormonal loss (e.g.vaginal dryness) may need treatment.
- Breast carcinoma risk increases with age.
- Hormone replacement therapy (HRT) lessens the unpleasant side-effects of the menopause, improves physical and psychological well-being and protects against postmenopausal osteoporosis. There may be an increased risk of uterine/ endometrial cancer.
- The male menopause (andropause) usually passes without major comment.
- All aspects of sexuality may continue into extreme old age.
- The ability to utilize a glucose load declines with increasing age.
- Thyroid function may be altered during illness — the 'sick euthyroid' syndrome.
- Thyroid function tests are a useful screening tool in unusual cases of ill health.

FURTHER READING

Buchsbaum HJ (ed.) *The Menopause*. Springer-Verlag, New York, 1983.

Burrows AW, *et al*. Thyroid hormones in the elderly sick. *Br Med J* 1975; 4:437–439.

Gosden RG. *Biology of the Menopause: The Causes and Consequences of Ovarian Ageing*. Academic Press, London, 1985.

Harman SM. Reproductive decline in men. In: Meites J (ed.), *Neuroendocrinology of Ageing*. Plenum Press, New York, 1983.

Hurley JR. Thyroid disease in the elderly. *Med Clin N Am* 1983; **67**:497–499.

Korenman SG (ed.). *Endocrine Aspects of Ageing*. Elesevier, New York, 1982.

11 THE AGEING ALIMENTARY SYSTEM

- Teeth
- Mucosa
- Oesophagus
- Stomach
- Small bowel
- Large bowel
- Motility
- Causes of constipation

Age-related changes occur in the gastrointestinal tract but function is usually maintained at a more than adequate level.

TEETH

Dental caries is responsible for the majority of tooth extractions in young people, but in the elderly periodontal disease is the main factor. Periodontal disease is accelerated by:

1. poor oral hygiene;
2. decreased production of saliva resulting from age changes in the salivary glands;
3. age atrophy of the alveolar bone with progressive exposure of the root surfaces and loosening of the teeth;
4. epithelial atrophy of the mucous membranes giving easily friable and traumatized surfaces.

Improved oral hygiene in the younger population should eventually lead to fewer dental problems, but currently the majority of elderly people are edentulous. In the edentulous the alveolar bone is resorbed and lower dentures especially will become loose. The use of dentures can pose significant problems, especially in institutions. Dentures should be marked and cleaned regularly. Problems with fit (poor speech or eating difficulties) should be referred early. Simple adjustments may be all that is necessary; however some problems may need specialist attention either by a general dental practitioner or one who has undergone postgraduate training specifically in the field of dentistry of the elderly.

MUCOSA

Leukoplakia appears as small white patches on the oral mucosa. It is associated with repeated mucosal trauma and may become malignant. Varicosities on the under-side of the tongue are seen in 40 per cent of elderly people. Their significance is unknown but attempts have been made to implicate vitamin C deficiency. Reduced saliva production predisposes to oral infections — especially ascending infection of the parotid gland producing septic parotitis.

OESOPHAGUS

This conveys food from mouth to stomach helped by peristaltic contractions. Primary peristaltic waves occur after swallowing and secondary waves arise when the upper oesophagus is distended by food. Sometimes a localized series of ring-like non-peristaltic contractions occur spontaneously. These tertiary contractions occur more frequently in the elderly and can produce symptoms of dysphagia (difficulty in swallowing).

In presbyoesophagus the normal swallow is not followed by a primary peristaltic wave. Instead non-propulsive contractions occur and there is incoordination in the lower oesophageal sphincter relaxing mechanism.

Clinically, diverticulae (pharyngeal pouches) can occur at the upper end of the oesophagus (more common in men and thought to be secondary to high pressure). Food may be aspirated from the pouch, and hence patients may present with dysphagia, coughing or repeated chest infections. Herniation of the lower oesophagus and upper part of the stomach (hiatus hernia) occurs in up to two-thirds of elderly people. The cause is probably muscular weakness around the diaphragmatic hiatus but constipation, straining, obesity and the wearing of corsets have all been implicated. Benign and malignant strictures are comparatively common.

STOMACH

Atrophic gastritis becomes more common in the elderly. The histological findings include decreased thickness of the gastric wall owing to atrophy of the mucosa and muscularis mucosae, infiltration with leucocytes, and loss of gastric glands. It is associated with an increased risk of pernicious anaemia (vitamin B_{12} deficiency) and gastric carcinoma. Gastric atrophy may produce achlorhydria. Pepsin activity is reduced whilst gastrin levels increase (correlated to the presence of antibodies to parietal cells). Gastric emptying appears delayed for fats but not for carbohydrates.

Gastric ulcers are more common in the elderly, especially the benign giant ulcer. Complications include haemorrhage, perforation and pyloric obstruction with higher mortality rates. Gastric carcinoma is also more common, possibly because its predisposing conditions (e.g. pernicious anaemia) are more frequent. Atypical 'silent' presentation of gastric ulcers include general debility, anorexia and weight loss.

SMALL BOWEL

The changes that occur here in normal ageing are quite subtle. Of clinical significance is that duodenal diverticulae occur and bacterial colonization can cause steatorrhoea (fatty stools). This is due to bile salt deconjugation by the bacteria leading to malabsorption (especially of iron, calcium, folate and B_{12}). The appendix gradually becomes involuted with age and appendicitis is rare. Age changes in the small intestine are small and their significance doubtful.

LARGE BOWEL

The large bowel and its nerve and blood supply is probably the part of the gut most affected by 'ageing'. The pathological consequences carry considerable mortality, morbidity and misery in the elderly. The colon receives liquid ileal contents, absorbs water, sodium and chloride, secretes potassium, bicarbonate and mucous and then stores faeces until evacuation.

Histological changes include an increase in connective tissue, atrophy of the muscle layer and arteriosclerosis. Colonic diverticulae increase with age in some populations (but not in those eating high-fibre diets).

MOTILITY

Eating food normally stimulates gut motility (the gastrocolic reflex) which is thought to be hormonal in nature. The response is increased by physical activity and there is poor gut motility in an immobile person whatever the age. This relationship between gut motility and physical activity is one of the main factors affecting constipation in the elderly. Using radio-opaque markers, or dyes, elderly people have been shown to have a slower gut transit time. Constipation is a term used frequently yet it can mean different things, such as a decreased frequency of bowel actions, the difficult passage of hard faeces or the increased retention of faecal material in the colon.

CAUSES OF CONSTIPATION

In the elderly there may be a combination of causes. (Table 11.1). The main complication of constipation is faecal impaction which can lead to:

1. faecal incontinence — impacted faeces act as a ball valve and liquid stool from higher up leaks around the faecal mass producing spurious diarrhoea;
2. intestinal obstruction (rarely perforation and peritonitis);
3. restlessness and agitation in the confused (BUT NEVER CAUSES CONFUSION);
4. retention of urine which may progress to overflow incontinence;
5. rectal bleeding due to mucosal ulceration

Table 11.1 Causes of constipation

Primary
1. Slow transit time aggravated by immobility
2. Incomplete emptying of the bowel due to poor muscle tone, unsatisfactory toilet arrangements or mental confusion
3. Diminished awareness of a loaded rectum, as in neurological disease
4. Ignoring the urge to defaecate owing to immobility, pain, confusion or poor toilet arrangements
5. Low bulk content arising from poor dentition or inadequate diet
6. Inadequate fluid intake

Secondary
1. Gastrointestinal disease (e.g. diverticular disease, carcinoma of colon or rectum, anorectal lesions such as fissures or haemorrhoids)
2. Hypothyroidism, hypercalcaemia
3. Drugs (e.g. morphine derivatives, iron and anticholinergics)

Carcinomas of the colon and rectum are common in the elderly, a rectal examination being mandatory as part of the routine examination. Benign polyps of the large bowel, familial polyposis coli and ulcerative colitis are recognized as premalignant conditions. Ischaemic colitis is common in the elderly, but because of good anastomotic channels, atheroma of the mesenteric vessels causes fewer problems than in the brain and peripheral circulation.

APPETITE AND NUTRITION

Appetite was thought to decline with age yet studies have shown that in those who reach extreme old age without impairment of physical and mental capabilities food intake is unchanged. Most reduction in appetite is secondary to acute or chronic disease processes compounded by social factors such as isolation, poor housing and poverty. Control of appetite (satiety and hunger) can be viewed as conditioned reflexes which are learned early in life and are continuously modified by external (environmental) and internal (homeostatic) mechanisms. There is only a small but continuous decline in basal metabolic rate after age 60. Hungry rats and humans prefer carbohydrate-rich foods as these are often readily absorbed and satisfy quickly. The elderly person living alone existing on a diet of sweet tea, jam sandwiches and chocolate is the classic example for the development of widespread deficiences. Beliefs about the likely wholesomeness of food on the basis of its appearance, colour, texture, smell and temperature are important in influencing appetite.

Meals are also social events and, apart from health problems and medication, the ambience of a meal may to some extent determine appetite and actual amounts of food eaten — hence the value of luncheon clubs and day centres for the isolated, lonely, recently bereaved and mildly confused.

The flavour of food is a combination of taste, texture, smell and temperature, but perception of taste and smell decline with age (and smoking). Sweet, sour and to a lesser extent bitter are gradually lost, though salt perception is only impaired much later. These facts may to some extent explain age differences in meal flavours and 'the young sweet tooth'. The elderly also take longer to eat a meal, so this is particularly important in institutions where food may be taken away before a person has finished and sub-optimal nutrition results. Anorexia is commonly seen as an acute symptom with infections, malignant disease, depression, alcohol abuse and as a side-effect of medication. It is also seen in severe dementia and post stroke.

Studies have shown that about 7 per cent of the elderly show clinical signs of malnutrition. There is undoubtedly a further group with subclinical malnutrition, only diagnosed when disease or stress causes their condition to become overt. A dietary history is therefore an integral part of the assessment of an elderly person. The major factors influencing nutrition are shown in Table 11.2.

Table 11.2 Major factors which influence nutrition

1. Ignorance: Elderly women of today learnt their cooking skills in a time of poverty and shortages. Elderly men may have never had to cook for themselves ('widower's scurvy')
2. Social isolation: The buying, preparing and eating of food is a social event (developed into an art in France), those living alone having a much poorer dietary intake
3. Physical disability: This may prevent people shopping, preparing and even eating food (e.g. rheumatoid arthritis, stroke)
4. Mental disturbance: Depression and confusional states can markedly affect nutrition
5. Iatrogenic: special diets ('gastric diet') are still being followed 40 years after a doctor advised them
6. Poverty: Existing on a state pension alone is equivalent to living on the poverty line. The elderly who can supplement their pension have been shown to have a better diet. In cold weather the choice may be between food or fuel and there is a close association between malnutrition and hypothermia
7. Impairment of appetite: By both emotional and physical causes
8. Dentition: Poor or absent dentition will alter a person's choice of diet (necessitating soft and mainly starchy foods)
9. Malabsorption: Common causes of malabsorption in the elderly are post gastric surgery, adult coeliac disease, pancreatic disease and bacterial overgrowth
10. Alcohol and drugs: With alcohol look for thiamine and folic acid deficiency
11. Increased requirements: Illness, pressure sores, infections and stress will all increase the requirements

Diagnosis. The diagnosis of deficiency states in the elderly can be difficult because symptoms and signs can be masked by disease. Biochemical and haematological investigations may help but can be misleading, in that the normal values quoted are all from medical students (not usually of retirement age and mostly male!). The most common deficiency states to be vigilant about are the anaemias (iron deficiency, folate deficiency), B_{12} deficiency (found in vegans), vitamin B complex deficiencies (riboflavin, niacin and pyridoxine), vitamin C (ascorbic acid) deficiency and vitamin D deficiency (osteomalacia). Vitamin C deficiency (scurvy) is very common subclinically (see Fig. 11.1).

Key points

- Periodontal disease is the main cause of teeth extraction.
- Currently the majority of elderly people are edentulous.

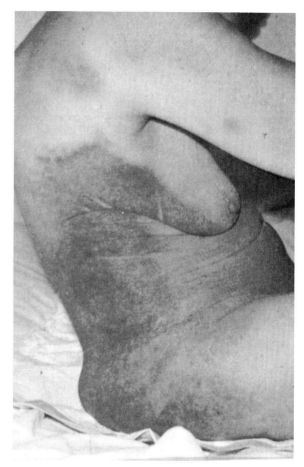

Figure 11.1 Sheet haemorrhage due to vitamin C deficiency

- Oesophageal problems (tertiary contractions, presbyoesophagus, pharangeal pouches, benign and malignant strictures) are common.
- Gastric ulcer may be symptomatic (haemorrhage, pain) or 'silent' producing general debility, anorexia and weight loss.
- Constipation is usually due to primary causes (decreased mobility, fluid intake and fibre) but can be due to secondary factors (e.g. hypothyroidism).
- Constipation never causes confusion.
- Appetite is unaffected in normal ageing.
- The flavour of food is a combination of taste, texture, smell and temperature but perception of taste and smell decline with age.
- Seven per cent of the elderly show clinical signs of malnutrition.
- Major factors which influence nutrition include ignorance, social isolation, physical and mental disability, poverty and illness.

FURTHER READING

Hellmans J, Vantrappen G (eds). *Gastrointestinal Tract*

Disorders in the Elderly. Churchill Livingstone, London, 1984.

Texter EC (ed.) *The Ageing Gut.* Masson, New York, 1983.

12 THE AGEING IMMUNE SYSTEM

- Humoral immunity
- Cellular immunity
- Autoimmune disease
- Tissue grafts
- Cancer

The age-related changes that occur in the immune system have been described as 'dramatic'. The subsequent immune dysfunction increases our susceptibility to infections, cancer and autoimmune disease. To function adequately the immune system is dependent upon numerous factors including histocompatability genes, hormonal changes, age, nutrition, antigen exposure and even psychological state.

The immune system has numerous component parts: bone marrow, lymph nodes, lymphatic vessels, the reticuloendothelial system, spleen and thymus. The cell types and secretory factors are listed in Table 12.1.

Table 12.1 Cell types and secretory factors

B lymphocytes
T lymphocytes
Monocytes
Granulocytes
Natural killer cells
Thymic factors
Lymphokines

isoantibody appear to decline with age, indicating deterioration in the B cell system (probably this is qualitative rather than quantitative). The primary antibody response, however, is also reduced in old age, and this may have clinical implications — there is an age-related rise in common infectious diseases.

HUMORAL IMMUNITY

Once the first two defence systems in the body are breached (skin/mucosa and phagocytic digestion by macrophages) the third line of defence against an infecting organism involves a humoral response. This involves an attack by specific antibodies secreted by mature B cells. Levels of natural antibody and

CELLULAR IMMUNITY

There is no obvious decrease in circulating lymphocyte numbers with age, but it is probable that T lymphocyte function deteriorates. It is well known that acquired delayed hypersensitivity reactions are reduced with age (anergy) as assessed by skin testing. The reaction should activate T-helper cells to release lymphokines, eventually causing localized tissue inflammation and destruction of the antigen. Anergy may have clinical significance in the reactivation of such diseases as tuberculosis and herpes zoster and in the clinical response to infections.

Macrophages appear to function normally in the elderly. Neutrophil function may be less good (seen clinically in the problem of severe staphylococcal infections in the elderly).

AUTOIMMUNE DISEASE

Some of the more common autoimmune diseases are listed in Table 12.2. A few appear to be related to age; for example, rheumatoid arthritis and autoimmune thyroiditis. In these conditions antibodies and/or T lymphocytes attack self-antigens. It appears that there is a genetic predisposition (via histocompatability genes), and hence some people will develop autoimmune disorders as they grow older.

Table 12.2 Autoimmune diseases

Addison's disease
Hashimoto's thyroiditis
Haemolytic anaemia
Myasthenia gravis
Pemphigus vulgaris
Rheumatoid arthritis

Although antibody production declines, autantibody production increases (nuclear antigens, immunoglobulin, and gastric parietal cell) with the aforementioned rise in autoimmune disease.

TISSUE GRAFTS

As a generalization there is less immune rejection of tissue grafts in the elderly (including organ transplants).

CANCER

As we age there is an increase in the number of cells that 'escape' normal growth and become cancer cells. At younger ages these abnormal cells are detected (probably via surface antigens) and are destroyed by macrophages, antibodies, T cells and natural killer cells. In the elderly two things occur which probably account for the increase in clinical cancer: there is the increase in cancer cell numbers, and surface antigens may be absent.

The thymus has a maturing effect on T lymphocytes in middle age and this declines with advancing years. Other lymphoid organs (gut lymphoid tissue, tonsils and appendix) get smaller with age. Stem cells (the precursors of lymphocytes) still replicate in old age but their function is impaired.

The above changes have specific clinical features but also more general implications. Some elderly people do not mount either a pyrexial response or a leucocytosis in the face of obvious infection. This may not be 'normal' ageing but is common enough to warrant mention. Studies have shown that if rectal rather than oral temperatures are taken more patients show a pyrexia, indicating that the site of temperature measurement may be more important than the underlying immune changes. It does mean, however, that treatment may need to be given if infection is suspected on clinical grounds before bacteriological confirmation and in the absence of some of the more common physical signs.

KEY POINTS

- To function adequately the immune system is dependent upon numerous factors, including histocompatability genes, age, nutrition and antigen exposure.
- Humoral immunity: levels of natural antibody decline with age, and there is a deterioration in the B cell system.
- Cellular immunity: T lymphocyte function deteriorates.
- Autoimmune disease increases with age. There is a genetic predisposition via histocompatability genes.
- There is less immune rejection of tissue grafts.
- The immune system is less effective in destroying cancer cells with advancing age.
- Some elderly people do not mount a pyrexial response or a leucocytosis in the face of obvious infection. Treatment should be given on clinical grounds before bacteriological confirmation.

FURTHER READING

Sternberg H. *Ageing of the Immune System.* In: Timiras P (ed.), *Physiological Basis of Ageing and Geriatrics.* MacMillan, New York, 1988.

13 THE AGEING PSYCHE

- Disengagement
- Use-it-or-lose-it
- Denial
- Losses
- Successful ageing

Psychological changes in old age are difficult to research because most studies are cross-sectional, comparing the attitudes and behaviour of people of different ages at the same point in time. When differences are found it is tempting to put them down to ageing, but it is clear that generational, or cohort, effects may be the cause. For example, it is well known that as we get older we become more preoccupied with our bowel function and more likely to take laxatives. Middle-aged people are very concerned about indigestion and frequently take anatacids, and young people subscribe to the value of fibre and vitamins to remain vital. These anxieties and behaviours reflect the eras in which successive generations grew up, and the prevalent medical concerns and advice given at different times.

Some of the cross-sectional data reinforce stereotypes and these enter into the dogma of the psychology of ageing. People stop having sex as they get older — true or false? The Kinsey Report, a cross-sectional study, found that 20 per cent of males were impotent at 65 years and 50 per cent at 75 years. However, a longitudinal study which followed men for six years

(admittedly only a short time) found only a small decline in activity. It is likely that if you start out sexually active, you will keep it up.

DISENGAGEMENT

One of the most popular theories of the psychology of ageing is disengagement. This theory grew out of the Duke University longitudinal studies of ageing. Investigators observed that those subjects with the highest life satisfaction (contentment, happiness) were those who had withdrawn from active engagement in social activities — the 'rocking chair' syndrome. It is unlikely that this method of growing old gracefully would suit everyone, and it probably reflects biases in the sample of volunteers studied; perhaps they were the only ones who were not too busy to answer the interviewers' questions.

USE-IT-OR-LOSE-IT

In contrast to disengagement, the 'use-it-or-lose-it' approach to ageing has great popular acclaim, and is a guiding principle in promoting a positive attitude. Evidence that physical capacity is maintained by regular activity is abundant. Whether psychological and other abilities are maintained by regular practice is uncertain, but it seems a reasonable assumption. Maintaining social engagement, learning new skills, making new friends, going on holidays are all things that a large number of better off old people do, and obtain great satisfaction in the process. Such approaches to encouraging involvement with others have to be tempered with a realization that the hearty 'joining in' spirit is not shared by everyone.

DENIAL

A mild denial of ageing is commonplace, and is promoted by the media in their 'keep young and beautiful if you want to be loved' youth image. Denial of some of the problems (e.g. financial, illness, bereavement) that accompany ageing can lead to an unwillingness to seek help, and for problems to get worse. People who adopt the denial strategy may battle on to maintain independence in the face of falling standards. In extreme cases they may fall into the Diogenes syndrome (see Chapter 27) with awful self-neglect.

LOSSES

Old age is a time of multiple losses; of job, status, partner, health, wealth and so on. This gloomy picture is central to the view of old age as a time of reflection on previous achievements to counterbalance the losses experienced. Surviving friends and relatives, coping with life's tragedies and experiencing its joys may be a source of inspiration; but with time they may be a cause of great unhappiness. Increasingly, older people become concerned about the need to leave something for their children and grandchildren, or to leave some record of their lives as part of the preparation for death. Death is one of the last taboos in our society, and many elderly people do not have opportunities to talk about those who have died ('Don't go on about him, you'll only upset yourself'), or indeed their own deaths. Many elderly people will talk very freely about death, even to comparative strangers.

The specific illness behaviours of older people are largely to do with impending death, and associated dependency on others. Older people may become overly health conscious, wanting every symptom checked out and becoming over-reliant on their doctors. Women who have been traditional care givers may find it much harder to accept a dependent role than men who have always 'suffered' with learned, socially sanctioned dependency on women!

SUCCESSFUL AGEING

A recent arrival on the psychology of ageing scene is the concept of achieving successful ageing through selection, adaptation and optimization of ability. An elderly person may be unable to carry out all the activities of daily living and social engagement of a younger person. Doctors, nurses, therapists and social workers have relatively stereotyped views of how old people should invest their energy and time. For example, maintaining continence is viewed as a worthwhile objective for the expenditure of energy. However, if a person has only a finite amount of energy (perhaps because of physical ill-health) it may make better sense to exhaust that energy through some other preferable activity; perhaps going to the pub. Consequently we should expect elderly people to select activities for themselves and not impose our own ideas on them.

Next a person may require help with achieving goals. This may require adaptation of the person's method of carrying out a task, or of the environment, or adaptation of the goal itself to make it more feasible. For example, the pub may have to come to the patient in hospital, rather than the patient to the pub. Optimization of ability refers to the practice required to achieve an adequate level of performance, and thus achieve the set goal.

The value of this theory of ageing is its wide applicability to the young old, the old old, and the oldest old. It also points a way for partners, relatives, friends and professionals to aid the process of successful ageing by emphasizing choices, the need to make priorities and to avoid stereotyped, repetitive lifestyles, particularly in institutions.

Perhaps the only certainty about the ageing psyche is that generalizations are imprecise, and heterogeneity is the rule.

Key points

- Cross-sectional studies are of very limited relevance in examining psychological aspects of ageing as the effects of both cohort and time period are likely to be marked. Such studies will tend to overestimate the true age-related changes: sexual activity is much less common in old men (from cross-sectional data), but sexually active old men are likely to remain active (longitudinal data).
- Disengagement theory states that elderly people gain contentment from withdrawing from active engagement — the 'rocking chair' syndrome.
- Use-it-or-lose-it theory is a more positive approach, suggesting that old people will gain most enjoyment (and feel better) if they keep up activities and learn new ones.
- Denial of ageing is a common defence mechanism, and may lead to failure to seek help when problems arise.
- Losses are commonplace in old age, but nonetheless a source of much sorrow. Many elderly people find comfort in talking about their losses, particularly of intimate partners.
- Successful ageing is the latest theory emphasizing the need to select activities, adapt to circumstances and optimize ability in the chosen activities.
- Psychological ageing is very variable and no single theory is adequate, but each may help explain the responses of some elderly people.

FURTHER READING

Baltes P, Baltes M. *Successful Ageing.* Cambridge University Press, Cambridge, 1990.

Kinsey AC, Pomeroy WB, Martin CE, *et al.* Sexual behaviour in the human male. Saunders, Philadelphia, 1948.

Martin CE. Factors affecting sexual functioning in 60–79 year old married males. *Arch Sex Behav* 1981; **10**:399–420

Murphy E, Brown G. Life events, psychiatric disturbance and physical illness. *Br J Psychiat* 1980; **136**:326–338.

Neugarten BN. Time, age and the life cycle. *Am J Psychiat* 1979; **136**:887–893.

PART TWO
ESSENTIAL MEDICINE
OF OLD AGE

14 THE HISTORY OF GERIATRIC MEDICINE

- The Poor Laws
- Workhouse life
- The birth of modern geriatric medicine
- Social or medical care?
- Types of service

Since the beginning of recorded medicine doctors have been interested in old age and its diseases. Pythagoras recorded the ages of man as childhood, youth, manhood and old age, and the most important of these was old age or the Gerocomice. Hippocrates (400 BC) wrote: 'Old men suffer from difficulty in breathing, catarrh accompanied by coughing, strangury, difficult micturition, pains at the joints, kidney disease, dizziness, apoplexy, cachexia, pruritus of the whole body, sleeplessness, watery discharges from the bowels, eyes and nostrils, dullness of sight, cataract, hardness of hearing.' In Roman times units for the care of old people were called 'gerocomia'. By 1000 AD the Arabian Avicenna (called the Prince of Physicians) outlined the care of the aged in his Canon of Medicine.

THE POOR LAWS

In medieval times the care of the sick (if it occurred at all) was based in religious institutions — mainly monasteries. Some religious orders in large premises (e.g. Tintern Abbey) built hospital wings and some monks became specialists in medical and nursing care. Later convents took on the caring/nursing role which in some centres continues to this day. Henry VIII, however, dissolved many of the monasteries in the sixteenth century, and later under Elizabeth I new laws were created to try to bridge the gap between alms/charity and vagrancy. The Elizabethan 'Poor Laws' were two Acts of Parliament passed in 1597 and 1601 specifically to keep the 'poor' off the streets and hence to discourage vagrancy (and its assumed concomitant lawlessness).

The Act of 1601 established a system of parish relief of the poor financed by compulsory 'poor rates' levied on property. The migrant poor remained a problem, so in 1662 an Act of Settlement defined that after 40 days residency the parish was liable for such a resident. The parish was chosen as the basic unit because the essential charitable nature of the law was meant to come from the community. This may have worked in rural areas but in towns and cities rich parishes often had the smallest dependent population and labour mobility ensured that work and home parishes were different. Initially the routine work (collecting rates and distributing relief) was carried out by churchwardens. This was supervised via the vestry meeting (an assembly of ratepayers), and at the county level by magistrates.

The Poor Law system designed for temporary unemployment and short-term sickness became the provider of care for the old, chronic sick, single-parent families (widows, deserted wives and unmarried mothers) and orphans. The infamous workhouses began appearing in the 1630s because the laws stated that the poor had to work in order to obtain relief. In 1722 Knatchbull's Act of Parliament was passed enabling all parishes to form voluntarily into unions to build workhouses and limit the amounts of relief given out. The aim was to encourage hard work, thriftiness and possibly limit family size, concepts born in the age of Adam Smith, only to be rediscovered in the 1980s. Not surprisingly a number of devices were tried to deter or uncover the potential fraudster, including legislation requiring 'paupers' to wear a badge with the letter 'P', and also published lists of relief receivers.

WORKHOUSE LIFE

By 1782 workhouses were renamed 'poorhouses' and acknowledged as asylums for the old and infirm. A few years later the ruling classes felt the ripples of fear from the French Revolution as discontent spread to the UK. Bread famines occurred and unemployment soared, resulting in numerous measures to keep order yet still provide meagre relief. The industrial revolution was beginning and with it more rural unemployment. Following the Napoleonic War reform was long overdue. A Royal Commission was set up and in 1834 the Poor Law Amendment Act was passed. It deliberately set out to stigmatize the poor and its catchphrase was 'less eligibility'. The regimen of the workhouse was harshened with men, women and children strictly segregated (exceptions being made for elderly couples of good character). Food was meagre (though presumably less awful than the diet of the destitute outside). The sick and elderly were given better rations. Work involved either laundry, cooking, stoking the boilers or tending the sick. Stonebreaking and oakum picking (separating the fibres of old ropes) were also part of this regimen. The giving out of alms continued ('out-relief') so that only about 20 per cent of Victorian paupers saw the inside of the poorhouse.

However, the aged and chronic sick provided the majority of the inmates.

Most workhouses developed an infirmary initially for the people who became ill suddenly, but the beds quickly became filled with the chronic sick and the disabled. Medical and nursing care were appalling and they soon developed a terrible reputation. The ill rich were visited in their own homes. Victims of accidents or those able to get 'sponsorship' via a wealthy subscriber were admitted to the voluntary hospitals (most of the major teaching hospitals in England came under this category). However, they were disinclined to take anything 'chronic' for fear of blocking the beds (and hence revenue) and would refuse admission of dubious cases. The parallel with some US practice and this re-emerging ethos in the UK health service is striking. By far the worst were the workhouse infirmaries (and their sister institutions the poor-law infirmaries). Conditions were so bad that campaigns were organized by the *Lancet* and Florence Nightingale and things gradually improved. Poverty surveys concerning the elderly by Booth and Rowntree helped educate and sway public opinion, but it was still necessary to wait for the Liberal reforms after the turn of the twentieth century before the provision of state pensions as a way out of poverty for the old became a reality.

THE BIRTH OF MODERN GERIATRIC MEDICINE

In France the term 'Gerocomie' was used to describe the need for a separate facility for the elderly. In America, Nascher in 1907 coined the word 'Geriatrics' (literally, old physician) to denote that branch of medicine dealing with the care of the aged. To live to be old, however, one must not die young, and at the turn of the century improvements in public health measures and better housing led to a dramatic decline in childhood mortality. The unequal access to medical care (financial and due to age) continued and the plight of the ill elderly was appalling. Within the midst of this degradation and sickness dedicated doctors taking an interest in the care of the elderly began to emerge. These luminaries founded what was later to be called Geriatric Medicine. Marjorie Warren as a newly qualified consultant in 1935 wrote powerful descriptions of the dreadful conditions awaiting her in the workhouse wards of the West Middlesex Hospital:

Having lost all hope of recovery with the knowledge that independence has gone, and with a feeling of helplessness and frustration, the patient rapidly loses morale and self-respect and develops an apathetic or peevish, irritable, sullen, morose and aggressive temperament which leads to laziness and faulty habits, with or without incontinence. Lack of interest in the surroundings, confinement to bed and a tendency to incontinence soon produce pressure sores, with the necessity for more nursing, of a kind that is appreciated by the patient. An increase of weight, especially the anterior abdominal wall, and an inevitable loss of muscle tone make for a complete bed-ridden state. Soon the well-known disuse atrophy of the lower limbs, with postural deformities, stiffness of joints and contractures completes the unhappy picture of human forms who are not only heavy nursing cases and a drag on society, but also are no pleasure to themselves and a source of acute distress to their friends.

The low status of the elderly became apparent during the Second World War when civilian casualties and wounded soldiers caused the aged sick to be evacuated into the workhouse wards. Complaints of neglect and under-treatment caused the Ministry of Health to set up an investigation which revealed a prevailing air of apathy about the care of the old. In contrast Dr Marjory Warren and a friend, Dr Trevor Howell, outlined a new basis for care indicating that the frail elderly and chronic sick could only be properly treated after taking a thorough history and performing a full examination, followed by what is now seen as the rudiments of the art/science of 'rehabilitation'. Treatable conditions were corrected and movement and muscle tone helped by standing exercises using the rails at the end of the bed. Wards were redecorated and painted and a system of remedial exercises for stroke patients was instituted in an atmosphere of hope, activity and cheerfulness. Patients with fractured femurs were operated upon and then mobilized early. The slogan 'bed is bad' became one of the basic mottoes of geriatric medicine. Geriatricians with long waiting lists started visiting those patients at home to assess and pre-empt complications — another milestone in care. Trevor Howell dealing with the Chelsea pensioners began research into the normal phenomena associated with normal ageing. This marked the start of Clinical Gerontology, the scientific study of ageing.

SOCIAL OR MEDICAL CARE?

Lord Amulree at the Ministry of Health (responsible for the aged and chronic sick) was impressed and saw the future: the new NHS taking responsibility not only for the chronic sick but also the frail elderly, managed by a new and developing breed of doctors — geriatricians. The argument that frailty in old age was often due to illness impressed him, and when the 1948 National Assistance Act was debated in Parliament he argued that the frail elderly should form part of the responsibility of the NHS, not of local government. He lost the vote and hence the frail old remained (under Part 3 of the Act) the responsibility of local govenment via Social Services to be housed in 'Part 3' homes. This was a poor outcome because he and the geriatricians were right and the difficulty remains to this day. Local authority residential homes are full of people placed there because of a perceived frailty; this has led to recent surveys showing that at least 50 per cent of residents are incontinent of urine and up to 75 per cent mentally confused. Frail? probably; sick? definitely. In the community and in hospitals are elderly people unable to find places in Part 3 homes, yet the homes are full of people who with earlier treatment may have continued to manage in their own home.

In 1947 Dr Howell and Lord Amulree founded the Medical Society for the Care of the Elderly, later to become the British Geriatrics Society. Through the Society and their personal teaching of interested doctors the specialty blossomed with national and international repercussions. Teaching hospitals founded Chairs in the subject, bringing in the first wave of teaching excellence to undergraduates; Professors Williamson, Exton-Smith, Isaacs and Brocklehurst to mention but a few. Their inspired revolution in both the medical, social and environmental aspects of health care led to enormous changes in bed, ward and even hospital management. Medical and nursing practices were challenged; for example, the use of tilt-back chairs and cot-sides were banned.

One area of care, the long-stay/continuing-care sector, remained a difficult backwater. The patients remained in poor accommodation with little or no medical and therapy input. The change in this state of affairs was largely helped by one man, Professor Peter

Millard. His constant fight to improve the quality of care, indeed the quality of life, for this group has led to this aspect being considered to have its own separate expertise and knowledge base, especially within the nursing and paramedical fields. His unit led the way in showing what was possible with dedication, imagination and humanity.

TYPES OF SERVICE

Health care of the elderly now has hundreds of consultants working closely with their counterparts in the psychiatry of old age. Different types of practice have emerged. In the *age-related service* admission usually depends on being over a chronological point (usually over 75 or even 85). This type of service has attracted many other specialists (e.g. gastroenterologists, chest physicians) into the field via posts which combine their specialty with 'an interest' in the elderly.

Appropriate-care services operate broadly on the needs of the patient, concentrating especially on rehabilitation, and hence do not admit all elderly people. The advantages and disadvantages of such systems are still being debated, the issues and arguments being complex.

A new era is in prospect. In a few years hospital-based continuing care (the starting point of the specialty) may cease to exist. The Conservative Government's decade of sponsored expansion of the private sector (and its financial penalizing of the NHS sector currently providing the care) spells its contraction and probable extinction. Independent Hospital Trusts and the emphasis on cost-effective health care will have unknown effects on the type of treatment the frail old will receive. Many assurances are given but they have to live up to the fact that currently for access, comprehensiveness and cost the NHS service for the elderly is the best and unrivalled in the world. Will that be the case in ten years time? Geriatric medicine

arose from the appalling neglect of the elderly in the workhouses; one hopes it will not be rediscovered in the residential and nursing homes of the future.

Key points

- The Elizabethan Poor Law system became the provider of care for the old and chronic sick.
- The workhouse and poorhouse infirmaries developed terrible reputations. This institutional stigma remains with elderly people to this day.
- The term 'geriatrics' was coined in the US by Nascher and literally means 'old physician'.
- Dr Marjorie Warren and Dr Trevor Howell helped found the specialty of geriatric medicine in this country.
- The 1948 National Assistance Act irrevocably split the 'sick' elderly (NHS) from the 'frail' (Social Services) — a split opposed by Lord Amulree on the advice of geriatricians.
- Standards of teaching, research and care rose with the appointment of the first 'wave' of academic specialists in geriatric medicine. Many medical schools now have Chairs in the specialty.
- Continuing care (long-stay care) requires the greatest skills and a high input of resources from professionals.
- The types of service provision are usually either age-related or appropriate-care.

FURTHER READING

Nascher IL. (1909) Geriatrics. *NY Med J* 1909; 21 August: 358–359.

Oxley GW. *Poor Relief in England and Wales 1601 – 1834*. David and Charles, London, 1974.

Rose ME. *The English Poor Law*. David and Charles, London, 1971.

Warren MW. (1946) Care of the chronic aged sick. *Lancet*; 1946; **i**:841–843.

15 THE ELDERLY IN SOCIETY

- Stereotypes and ageism
- Demography
- Heterogeneity of elderly people
- Care in the community
- Institutional care

STEREOTYPES AND AGEISM

The very phrase 'the elderly' evokes an image in the mind: frail, confused, little old ladies, some of them nice like your granny, some of them not. Many other social groups experience stereotyping in society — ethnic minorities, homosexuals, professional groups, trade unionists — partly because this is a means for

Table 15.1 The stereotyped view of old people

Old people:
- need similar services
- are of little value
- are a burden on society
- are slow to accept change
- cannot look after themselves
- are deaf and need to be shouted at
- are sweet
- are like children

people to cope with their ignorance and deal with people they may fear. Stereotyping helps people to make sense of society, and their place in it. The phenomenon will not disappear, but advocates of elderly people (including elderly people themselves, as well as professionals) have a duty to ensure that some of the adverse consequences of stereotyping are reduced. Stereotypes lead to prejudice; this is *ageism* (see Table 15.1).

The last four decades have been a period of growth and reconstruction following the Second World War. The major emphasis has been on young people — our future — often at the expense of the other end of the age spectrum. Society has become well-geared to the needs of young people because they are a major economic force, spending large amounts of money. Moreover youth culture, young looks and ideals have often been promoted by advertising agencies and the mass media.

The 1990s have seen the dawning of a realization that young people are getting scarcer: school rolls are falling in many parts of the UK; and the demand for young people in the workplace (particularly in health and social services) far exceeds supply. By contrast, there are more old people around, and some of them

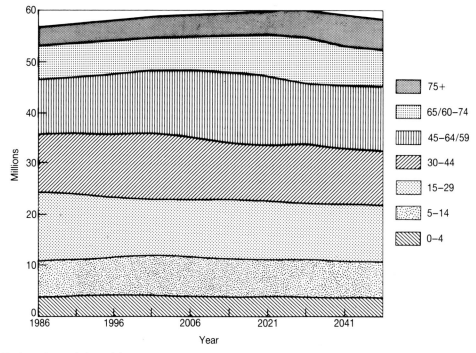

Figure 15.1 Projected population of the UK

have relatively large amounts of money to spend — they are now an economic force to be considered by the market. (This is now reflected in the Paris fashion shows which feature many male and female models over 60 years old).

In the USA, the 'greying of America' has been associated with a new wave of militancy amongst elderly people — the Grey Panthers! Elderly people have campaigned vigorously to ensure that politicians do not ignore the fact that they have needs which should be met by society, and that they have paid taxes longer than most. From the political standpoint a key issue is that they have a lot of votes to contribute during elections.

DEMOGRAPHY

Remarkable changes in the age structure of the population have occurred over the last century, and there have been two major forces: reductions in fertility, and declines in infant mortality (not from better health care, but from socio-economic development). These forces are discussed in Chapter 1.

The number of old people has risen from about 2 million in 1901 to around 10 million in 1991. Census figures since 1971 are shown in Table 15.2. But what do we mean by 'old people'. Old age can be a long time

— many people now survive into their high 80s, or even 90s, so old age may last as long as 20 to 30 years (as long as many reading this text have been alive!). It is necessary to split the elderly up into smaller age groups to see what has been happening to them over the last few decades.

Table 15.2 Pensioners* in Britain (Millions)

	1971	1981	1991	2001
All ages	54.4	54.8	55.2	56.0
60+/65+	8.9	9.8	10.1	9.9
Percentage	16.4	17.9	18.3	17.7

* Women 60+, Men 65+.

Census figures are also used to predict what will happen in the future — population projection (see Fig. 15.1). Prediction is a risky business; but provided there are no world wars, or life-threatening epidemics, and we are not too ambitious in predicting the future too far ahead, predictions can give good guidance to what will happen. On the other hand, planners have been less good at doing anything about the demographic predictions.

HETEROGENEITY OF ELDERLY PEOPLE

'Heterogeneity' is derived from two Greek words: *heteros* meaning 'other' and *genos* meaning 'kind'. We

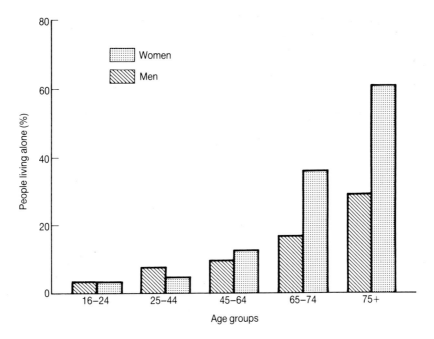

Figure 15.2 People living alone in Britain in 1988

use the term to mean 'made up of diverse kinds of people'. Old people are simply young people who have lived for a longer time than others. The idea of being a *pensioner* has led to chronological age (the number of years lived) being used to define 'old age'. We tend to think of the elderly as those people over 60 or 65 years. Such a definition is, of course, arbitrary.

It is useful to think of old people in three distinct groups: the young old (65 to 74), the old old (75 to 84), and the oldest old (85+). The social and biological characteristics of people in each of these age groups is sufficiently distinct to make these categories meaningful. For example, the young old are recently retired, tend to be wealthier than other elderly people, and often provide much of the care for the oldest old. By contrast the oldest old were born at the turn of the century, many of the women never married, or lost husbands in world wars. They went through the economic slump of the 1930s, and have tended to be poor, and live in old, unmodernized houses. They are much more likely to be disabled by physical and mental illness, and to live alone (see Fig. 15.2).

CARE IN THE COMMUNITY

Most old people want to live in their own homes and fortunately the vast majority do. The present community care legislation in the UK (the National Health Service & Community Care Act 1990) tends to make us think that community care is something new. It is not, and services to allow elderly people to live in their own homes have been around for a very long time.

The services that are offered fall into six main categories: relatives and friends (informal carers); local authority social services; local health services; independent (i.e. private and voluntary) sector services; local housing department services; and the central government department of social security. The characteristics of each of the services are very different, as is the range of services on offer. Informal carers are always available and will inevitably have to carry out whatever task needs doing, regardless of time of day, or skill required to do the job properly. By contrast, statutory agencies tend to provide much more circumscribed services, and disputes over who does what are increasingly common as services come under increased pressure.

Table 15.3 shows the main services provided by different agencies. With so many providers it is sometimes difficult to work out who should do what, and who will pay for what. In part, this is what the community care legislation hopes to simplify. For example, the dispute over who should bathe an elderly person — district nursing services or local authority home care services — has led to no baths at all in some areas. The task has now been redefined as 'social bathing' to put it firmly into the hands of the local authority services.

Table 15.3 Some of the services provided for elderly people

Informal carers
Personal hygiene
Domestic tasks
Nursing tasks
Financial help
Counselling
Almost anything!

Local authority social services
Home helps
Meals on wheels
Part 3 homes
Social worker
Good neighbour schemes
Adult fostering
Respite care
Occupational therapy
Day centres
Lunch clubs

Local health services
Family doctor: treatment, 75+ screening
Hospital beds
Home nursing
Out-patients
Pharmacist
Therapists
Chiropody
Dietitian

Private services
Institutional beds
Private nursing
Limited home care services

Voluntary services
Crossroads
Age Concern projects
Good neighbour schemes
Lunch clubs
Day centres
Residential homes

Community care legislation. Although the new Act was due to come into effect in 1991, it has been delayed to 1993. The major change is that local authority social service departments will take the leading responsibility for planning and monitoring of care for elderly (and disabled) people. Local authorities are also major providers of services to elderly people, but it is intended that the independent sector should take a much greater part in providing basic services like meals, home helps and respite care in the future. A further change is that individual clients will no longer get a 'take it or leave it' package of services, but will be assessed, will have a care plan, and the impact of services will be monitored.

Furthermore, many statutory services will have to be paid for directly by the user.

INSTITUTIONAL CARE

Institutional care is provided in three main settings: the local authority residential homes (under Part 3 of the National Assistance Act 1948); the hospital long-stay wards; and the 'independent' sector — private residential and nursing homes, and 'not-for-profit' housing association residential homes (see Figs. 15.3 and 15.4). A small number of specialist homes exist; examples are homes for elderly actors, for elderly seamen, and Jewish homes. These are usually run on a charitable basis.

These institutions have certain informal rules for selection of appropriate clients. In general, Part 3 homes and residential homes will take clients who are independently mobile (with or without aids), who can dress themselves, and who are continent of urine and faeces. Some will not take patients with dementia syndromes if there are associated behaviour problems (e.g. wandering or biting). Residential homes are not staffed by nurses, but by care attendants, and do not have sufficient staff or equipment to look after very dependent people. Nursing homes must have at least one trained nurse on the staff, but in practice the bulk of the care is provided by untrained care assistants. Nursing homes have variable selection criteria, and there is increasing evidence that private homes are taking fewer severely disabled patients than the hospital long-stay wards. This is not surprising since disabled people cost more to manage well, which eats into profit margins.

A major difference between long-stay hospital care and other institutional care is that the former is free! Consequently there can be conflict in deciding who should have a free hospital long-stay bed and who should have to use their own resources. Escalating costs in the private sector may preclude all but the relatively wealthy from going into a private nursing home.

It might be argued that the uncontrolled growth of private residential and nursing homes, subsidized by the public purse, was one of the main forces leading to the change in community care organization. It is a good example of how 'free markets' can lead to growth that is neither desirable (most people do not want to be in institutions) nor cost-effective. Of course, 'the market' was not really a free one. Central government

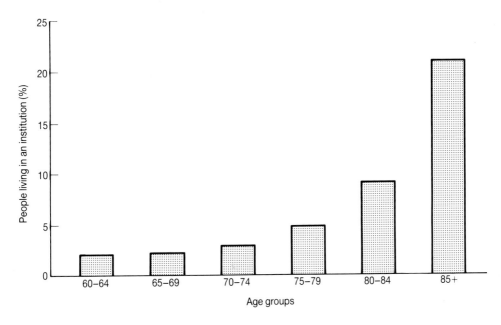

Figure 15.3 People living in institutional care in London in 1981 (taken from census data); about 4 per cent of pensioners live in institutions

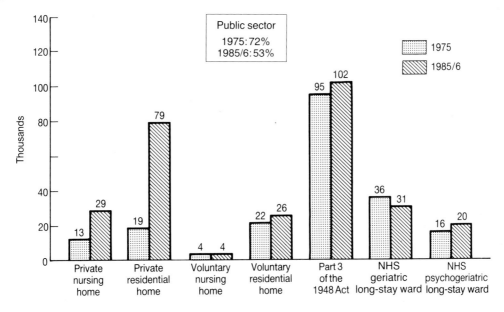

Figure 15.4 Elderly people in long-term care in England, 1975 to 1985/86 (Laing, 1988)

funds are available to people wishing to go into private residential and nursing home care. The cost rose from £10 million in 1979 to £1 billion in 1989.

Surprisingly, no health or social assessments are required before an individual goes into a private home (unlike local authority homes and hospital long-stay care), and only rudimentary systems of registration and monitoring are set up. Consequently standards in such homes are very variable (although standards in the state sector, too, are variable). A major problem for residents presently in such private homes is that their money is running out. Costs have increased dramatically, but central government grants have failed to keep pace with this, leaving elderly people to rely on the generosity of their families and charitable trusts. Some have even found themselves thrown out, and only admission to hospital then prevents them being literally on the street.

No amount of community care will stop some elderly people requiring institutional care, particularly the oldest old, living alone. A society that does not provide for such needs has ceased to care.

Key points

- Stereotypes of old age and old people are common and may be disadvantageous.
- The demographic changes are best classified into age bands: young old (65–74), old old (75–84), and oldest old (85+). The numbers of the oldest old will increase dramatically over the next 30 years.
- Care in the community is provided by many different agencies: informal carers; social services; health services; housing departments; the inde-

pendent sector. Each agency has a different range of services, operates under different constraints, and with a different philosophy.
- However much community care is provided for elderly people, a small number will require institutional care. Without this back-up, community care will not work.
- The growth in private sector nursing and residential homes has been extraordinary. The social security bill has grown from £10 million in 1979 to £1 billion in 1989.

FURTHER READING

Caring for People: Community Care in the Next Decade and Beyond. HMSO, London, 1989.

Fennel G, Phillipson C, Evers H. *The Sociology of Old Age.* Open University Press, Milton Keynes, 1988.

Wells N, Freer C (eds). *An Ageing Population: Burden or Challenge.* Macmillan, London, 1988.

16 SOCIAL NETWORKS

- Informal and formal social networks
- Requirements for a successful support system
- Anatomy of social networks
- Psychology of the social network

The emphasis in the training of health care workers, and medical students in particular, is upon disease, because the detection, investigation, treatment and prevention of disease is the justification for medicine, its one specific function. Much of the teaching is inevitably in large hospitals where staff and facilities can be readily available and deployed to greatest advantage; but it is important, given the nature of the diseases prevalent in the developed countries in the 1990s and the state of medicine there, that students should see disease from a wider perspective. Disease even when detected and treated often leaves disabilities. The majority of frail and disabled people including those with severe functional impairments live in private households. To do so they depend to a greater or lesser extent upon those who constitute their social networks — informal and formal. A knowledge of the anatomy and psychology of social networks is important.

INFORMAL AND FORMAL SOCIAL NETWORKS

Any person can be regarded as being at the centre of and interacting with a series of subsystems of people. These subsystems usually operate independently of one another, but they occasionally intersect, and this is particularly the case when there is disability and at a time of crisis.

The informal network

The informal network of support consists of kin (nuclear and extended family), friends and neighbours. The informal primary group is usually small in size and has a long history of contact with the old person, contact which may have been rewarding, hostile or mixed. There may have been emotional bonds and a more or less pronounced sense of commitment. It may have less skill than the formal network but it has the great advantage of availability at all times (usually), of being able to deal with unexpected events and emergencies, of being flexible and unencumbered by professional and other demarcation boundaries. Finally there are the virtues of familiarity and continuity. In contrast the formal agencies can draw on a potentially larger pool of people and they possess a range of technical expertise, skill and resources which may be essential for the patient.

The formal network

The formal network of support consists firstly of the basic financial entitlements available to the elderly (e.g. retirement and supplementary pensions, attendance allowance). Then there are the statutory agencies which carry out the economic and social policies of central and local government, but actually provide the services: the National Health Service (general practitioner, district nurse, health visitor, etc.) and the local authority Social Services department (social worker, home help, meals on wheels, day centre). Finally there are the voluntary or quasi-formal organizations which are independent of government but often encouraged and supported financially by it (e.g. Age Concern, Help the Aged, MIND).

REQUIREMENTS FOR A SUCCESSFUL SUPPORT SYSTEM

There are three major requirements for a social network to act as a successful support system:

1. Socialization;
2. The carrying out of tasks needed in every-day living;
3. Assistance in illness or crisis.

To a considerable extent the informal network is sufficient for those needs. In a survey of elderly people living in a large inner city it was concluded that kin are clearly considered the primary source of help, regardless of the task. Only to the extent that family, particularly children, are not available do friends, neighbours and formal organizations become important in the provision of social support.

ANATOMY OF SOCIAL NETWORKS

No assessment of an older person with even slight disability is complete without a description of those people available to help. The enumeration must be systematic and should include the following particulars.

Informal networks

Names, addresses, telephone numbers and frequency of contacts with relatives, neighbours and friends. The nature of tasks undertaken for or on behalf of the patient should be listed.

Formal networks

Specific enquiry should be made about contact with the people and services listed in Table 16.1. The tasks undertaken and the frequency of involvement should be specified in detail.

Table 16.1 Anatomy of the formal network

Domiciliary services	
1. General practitioner District nurse Health visitor Community psychiatric nurse	The primary health care team
2. Social worker Home help/home care Meals on wheels	Social Services: Field workers
3. Sitting services Visiting schemes	Often via voluntary groups
Institutional services	
4. Hospitals Day hospitals (medical/psychiatric)	NHS
5. Day centres Luncheon clubs Old peoples homes	Social services and independent residential and day care

In practice it is surprising how much input rather than how little there is in the care of an elderly person. Much of it, however, is often uncoordinated and unplanned. Part of the art of medicine is to visualize the person in their world rather than *in vacuo* or only in relation to one's own agency and then, as far as possible, to plan care jointly. The people partaking have their own attitudes and needs in relation to the patient and these views must be obtained. If necessary a case conference should be convened inviting all concerned in the person's care.

PSYCHOLOGY OF THE SOCIAL NETWORK

There are a great variety of feelings, attitudes and views held about frail and disabled old people, not solely by their families, friends and neighbours but also by professionals. In the assessment of what can be done to help the person these feelings may count for much more than marginal abnormalities in physical test results and may be as important as specific treatment. They must be recognized and channelled in support of the patient. For example, by helping the carer directly the patient may be helped indirectly.

Anxiety in the network may be constructive in moderate degrees but destructive if unjustified or excessive. It may be the latter because of:

1. ignorance of the facts surrounding the patient's illness as a result of communication barriers;
2. the patient is viewed as a burden which is unshared;
3. difficulty in accepting the lowered standards which may be inevitable with disability;
4. concern over risk;
5. the fear of threat or criticism towards a carer should the patient come to harm.

Much can be done to reduce anxiety by listening, by allowing 'ventilation' to take place, by explanation and by jointly considering the possible steps to be taken. All too often barriers are erected by professionals where what is required is a sense of partnership between them and the supporters for the client's benefit. Depression in carers can be alleviated by reducing their burden through partial relief from total care, by psychological support and sometimes by medication.

Guilt may be a major problem. The person's behaviour may cause irritation, leading to outright hostility, rejection or even violence. Occasionally it can lead to a mixture of emotions (ambivalence) in which the negative features may be masked by intense compensations or reaction formation in which there is apparent excessive devotion concealing the resentment.

The point to bear in mind is that such so-called psychodynamic factors always exist in relation to disabled people, whatever the disability and whatever the age of the patient. They must be understood and then they can be handled constructively by those with empathy, counselling skills and the willingness and ability to spend time. Many carers and patients would benefit from the support of more skilled counselling were it available. Self-help groups and large organizations like the Alzheimer's Disease Society and the Parkinson's Disease Society can give invaluable support.

People under stress turn first to their nearest and dearest, who provide most of the care for disabled people. It is never enough to view a person in isolation, let alone to be concerned only with the disease. Illness in one person inevitably has repercussions on those in their social environment. To help the client most, once everything possible has been done for the disease process, management must be planned for the carers as well as for the person.

Key points

- The majority of frail and disabled people (including those functionally impaired) live in their own homes.
- Support subsystems can be classified into formal and informal.
- Formal networks include financial entitlements, the statutory agencies and the voluntary sector.
- Informal networks include family/relatives, friends and other close carers.
- Successful support systems must help carry out the tasks needed in daily living, assist in illness or crisis and help in socialization.
- No assessment is complete without a full description of informal and formal networks.
- In times of crisis people turn to their nearest and dearest.

FURTHER READING

Abrams M. *Beyond Three Score and Ten: A Second Report on a Survey of the Elderly.* Age Concern, London, 1980.

Stevenson O. *Age and Vulnerability: A Guide to Better Care.* Age Concern, London, 1989.

Townsend P. *The Last Refuge.* Routledge and Kegan Paul, London, 1962.

Townsend P. *The Family Life of Old People.* Routledge and Kegan Paul, London, 1987.

17 PRESENTATION OF DISEASE

- Delay
- Atypical presentation
- Multiple pathology
- Social presentation
- Teamwork
- Social networks
- The environmental revolution

Even for the lay person there are some disease processes that are immediately recognizable by their presentation. An adult complaining of crushing central chest pain that goes down his left arm, leaving him sweating, breathless and nauseated, is likely to provoke the alarm bells of 'heart attack' and get the appropriate response. This pattern recognition of symptoms and signs is obviously enhanced to a fine art during medical training, so that conditions less common than myocardial infarction result in the same process — history, examination and diagnosis. Thus there is a traditional pattern of disease presentation in younger people that even if not articulated well results in an 'I am sick — help me' scenario.

Two major factors influence the recognition of disease processes in the elderly: acceptance of ill-health with a subsequent delay in seeking help, and the atypical presentation of disease processes.

DELAY

Acceptance of ill health as 'ageing' and the resulting disabilities mean that many elderly people expect to be frail and rarely complain or seek help at an early stage. Dramatic complaints (severe pain, vomiting blood, etc.) may still elicit the traditional response but less life-threatening episodes can be accepted as change and part of the ageing process. This picture is especially noticeable in inner city areas with their poor history of primary health care and where health expectations (especially amongst the elderly) are low. Coming to terms with some disability/change is necessary at all ages and acceptance is part of successful survival. However, the tacit acceptance of deterioration in, for example, eyesight, hearing, teeth and feet as part of the inevitable ageing process may lead to treatable conditions being ignored and independence being lost.

ATYPICAL PRESENTATION

The pioneers in the field of health care of the elderly outlined some fundamental differences in disease presentation, simple in themselves and yet laying the foundation to one of the most complex branches of

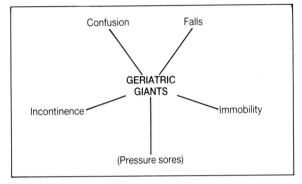

Figure 17.1 Geriatric giants

medicine. This fact of atypical presentation, understanding the concept and acting on it is so profound as to border on being one of the most essential elements for a student and practitioner to comprehend. It is the starting point for good health care for the elderly.

The term 'geriatric giants' (see Fig. 17.1) was coined by Professor Isaacs. It refers to the 'pattern recognition' of a set of symptoms and signs that may have as their cause *any* disease process. Diseases as different in aetiology as pneumonia, myocardial infarction, urinary tract infection or drug toxicity can present classically or as one of the giants. This pattern

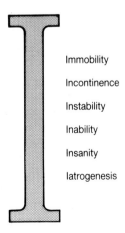

Immobility

Incontinence

Instability

Inability

Insanity

Iatrogenesis

Figure 17.2 The I's of old age

of presentation has been refined and expanded, and another *aide-mémoire* is shown in Fig. 17.2.

A useful analogy is a 'fit' in a child. This is only a symptom and does not imply a diagnosis, which could be a febrile illness, epilepsy, meningitis, drugs, etc. Health professionals would never dream of labelling fits as 'childhood events'. In the same way neither should falls or incontinence be treated as an 'ageing process'. Look beyond the presenting symptom and find the disease behind.

In most cases alleviation of symptoms and treatment of disease will be possible. In some the disease process will not be cured but these will be a minority. Not responding correctly to the atypical presentation is not only an intellectual failure but is also profoundly detrimental to the patient and leads to an enormous waste of resources.

There are two other important aspects concerning the altered presentation of disease in old age. One is the concept of multiple pathology being present in many elderly people and the other is the recognition of the 'social' presentation of disease and the response that subsequently occurs.

MULTIPLE PATHOLOGY

The altered presentation of disease in the elderly is often secondary to more than one disease process in the individual. They may be causally linked; for example, confusion secondary to hypoxia due to heart failure caused by ischaemic heart disease. Typically they are not, and it is common to have a medical 'problem list' consisting of falls secondary to osteoarthrosis of the knees, plus a contribution from onychogryphosis, 1° hypothyroidism, hiatus hernia, macular degeneration giving poor vision (making self-medicating and drug compliance further problems). The art is in trying to identify and treat the most important underlying problems and, using a multi-disciplinary approach, find ways of compensating for as many of the other deficits as possible.

SOCIAL PRESENTATION

It has been widely accepted (since the Poor Laws of the sixteenth century) that medicine has nothing to do with social problems. This is manifestly untrue for disease at any age leads to concomitant social and psychological upheaval. The holistic approach in health care of the elderly recognizes this; indeed, 'social admission' should be the sixth basic geriatric giant. 'Social admission' is currently a perjorative term in a hospital setting. It actually indicates a lack of history-taking and examination that should have uncovered a disease process resulting in the 'social' response. The response may be that of exhausted relatives leaving a person in Casualty, or neighbours calling a social worker or police to 'do something'. Many patients are actually barred admission and referred to Social Services for 'appropriate' admission to an old people's home and the inappropriate cycle is established. This results in ill elderly people in social care (when they should be in hospital) and those in need of 'care' in hospital or at home denied access.

The recognition of the social presentation of disease means that some doctors have now been trained to rush towards rather than away from social problems. The traditional medical behaviour of history-taking and examination then leads to the identification of multiple problems. Investigation of and solutions to these problems require modern investigating techniques and treatments. Departments of Health Care of the Elderly with beds in District General Hospitals have access to these facilities and can provide a diagnostic and treatment service. The problems of limited resources means that conflict with professional colleagues can develop. Manifestations of this discord include the use of the term 'bed blocker' and the refusal to admit 'social problems' by some clinicians, and on the other hand the development of a strict age related discipline by some geriatricians.

The learning curve of the pioneers in the field incorporated the problems of delay in diagnosis, atypical presentation, the role of multiple pathology and 'social' presentation. They developed a framework to cope with these problems and set the basis for the holistic approach that is the hallmark of health care for the elderly in the UK. Elements of this framework were the development of teamwork, the recognition of social networks and the environmental revolution.

TEAMWORK

Multiple problems require staff trained to deal with them or teamwork by staff trained to deal with individual problems. The range of people and their skill mix brought together to help solve client/patient problems is considerable (see Chapter 42). No one model of multidisciplinary working has achieved prominence and the practice is not always straightforward or without criticism. Inherent in teamwork is some level of conflict: when faced with a difficult task each member of the team may suggest a different solution. Successful teamwork therefore requires leadership if anything is to be achieved.

If the team objective is set as rehabilitation and discharge then the team will consider it has failed if it does not resettle people at home or elsewhere. Such resettlement requires the development of methods of aftercare to ensure successful discharge.

SOCIAL NETWORKS

There is no such thing as independence because everyone is dependent upon others to some extent. Rather there is relative acceptance and tolerance. There are some general patterns to the social network around each individual, but each network is different and to understand disease in old age it is essential that the social network is studied. This network can be simplistically divided into formal and informal (see Chapter 16). The formal consists of the statutory services, which are comprehensive but somewhat inflexible in timing and frequency. Informal networks (family, friends, carers and neighbours) are not professional but are flexible and usually infinitely more available at unsocial hours.

Each social network is unique to an individual. Requests come to others for help when the tolerance levels of the networks change and acceptance changes to rejection. The point at which rejection occurs is dependent upon inherent strengths and weaknesses of the individuals or systems in the network. Some want help early, some too late and some not at all. An outline of a person's social network prior to admission and after discharge is an important ingredient of our knowledge concerning them.

THE ENVIRONMENTAL REVOLUTION

The fundamental new knowledge base of a consultant caring for the elderly is based upon an attack on prolonged bed rest. This has led to the refurnishing of wards with beds of adjustable height and without cot-sides (for they are not necessary if the bed is low) and chairs of variable height.

Not all changes have been beneficial, with the unacceptable restraint of bed-rest having been swapped for the tilt-back chair or chair with restraining table or restraining belt. In the modern ward for the elderly, people are now nursed in bed only when sick, and up and dressed in their own clothes in the stage of rehabilitation. An environmental revolution has taken place that needs to be recognized and understood.

| Key points |

- Many elderly people accept ill-health as normal ageing and delay in seeking help.
- Disease processes in old age usually present atypically.
- The 'geriatric giants' consist of confusion, falls, immobility, incontinence and pressure sores.
- The elderly often have more than one disease process (multiple pathology).
- The atypical presentation of illness often leads to an erroneous label of 'social problem'.
- Multidisciplinary teamwork is an essential element to the holistic approach to care of the elderly.
- Social networks consist of formal and informal groupings.
- Hospital environments have to be 'user-friendly' if rehabilitative results are to be achieved — the concept of the environmental revolution.

FURTHER READING

Abrams M. *Beyond Three Score and Ten: A Second Report on a Survey of the Elderly.* Age Concern, London, 1980.

Isaacs B, Livingstone M, Neville Y. *Survival of the Unfittest.* Routledge and Kegan Paul, London, 1972.

18 HISTORY-TAKING AND EXAMINATION: HELPING YOUR ELDERLY PATIENT TO HELP YOU

- The GP consultation
- Meeting a patient for the first time
- Positioning, vision and hearing
- The environment
- Getting the story
- The confused patient
- Activities of daily living
- A drug history
- Corroboration of the evidence
- Examination
- 'Extras' for the elderly
- Explanation and reassurance

Whether you are a doctor, a nurse, a therapist, a social worker, a student, or a carer you will sometimes have to obtain information from an elderly person. Sources of difficulty can come from the information giver, the information taker, and the environment. It is all too easy to blame the elderly person, and it is commonplace to see comments like 'rambling old buffer' or 'difficult, vague historian'. Such remarks written in case notes (and they are more often seen in doctors' notes than in those of any other professional group) tell us more about the attitudes and behaviour of the history-taker than the patient.

Fig. 18.1 can be looked upon as a summary of the crucial aspects of history-taking to be discussed in this chapter.

THE GENERAL PRACTITIONER CONSULTATION

Much of the discussion in this chapter assumes a hospital or outpatient setting, but is just as relevant in a GP's surgery.

In general practice, history-taking is spread over months and even years as a mutual process of 'getting to know you' occurs. This is one of the strengths of general practice because it allows the doctor to interpret the patient's present symptoms in the light of previous encounters. The ability to do this is greatly improved by a structured case record with a problem list and a prescribing card. These should be reviewed prior to any consultation so that the present problem can be fitted rapidly into an overall picture of the patient.

TAKING A MEDICAL HISTORY

- The introduction

- Timing, interest

- Position and comfort

- Vision, hearing, cognition

- Environment

- Use of multiple sources

- Interview versus interrogation

Figure 18.1 Taking a medical history

The nature of the patient's presenting complaint must be sorted into potentially serious (e.g. chest pain, breathlessness, vomiting); might be serious (e.g. general aches and pains, weakness, a fall); probably not serious (e.g. a dizzy spell, feeling 'out of sorts', sore throat). Action may be decided at this stage for the potentially serious category. However, for most patients the key point to be established at the outset is whether there has been any deterioration in the patient's functional ability. Has she stopped doing the shopping? Is she unable to do the heavy housework? Has she lost interest in things generally? Further enquiry should be about other 'geriatric giants' — especially incontinence, falls and confusion (see

Chapter 17).If there has been no change in performance of activities of daily living and none of the common presentations of occult disease, then the GP can use time to make the diagnosis. This means reviewing the patient in a week or so to decide whether the symptoms are progressing or not, and whether new problems have arisen.

It is worth remembering that about 70 per cent of people aged over 80 years have some degree of disability, and in 20 per cent this will be severe. Age is quite a useful yardstick to determine how intensively to treat a problem. Very old people are much more vulnerable to sudden deteriorations. A 'mild' chest infection in an 85-year-old can rapidly turn into a fall with associated hip fracture, whereas in a 70-year-old this is much less likely. In general, early and aggressive treatment is likely to be rewarded by fewer complications.

To provide adequate assessments of elderly people in general practice is not easy. It requires a willingness to commit sufficient time to history-taking and examination — usually best done by seeing those patients who appear, during a short appointment, to have a potentially serious problem again for a fuller assessment of at least 30 minutes. Unless this is done the familiarity that is such a useful tool in general practice can become the enemy of older patients. Furthermore, it is no sign of incompetence or idleness to refer patients for a comprehensive assessment to the local department of health care of the elderly. Consultants have more time to spend with patients, and have the resources of other professionals to draw upon. All too often problems of incontinence (both urinary and faecal), depression, Parkinsonism, myxoedema, episodes of left ventricular failure, and many more have been going on for months or years before they are recognized and treated.

MEETING A PATIENT FOR THE FIRST TIME

The introduction is crucial to what follows. A cheerful 'How are you doing, grandpa?' is unlikely to be greeted with much enthusiasm by a retired bank manager you have never met before. Introductions should be straightforward, relatively formal, and should respect the dignity of the person. Eye contact, a greeting, an outstretched hand (expecting a returned handshake), your name, and the purpose of your visit are all that are required to get started.

Eye contact is the first step. Can the person see you? Does he smile in response to your smile? Does he look perplexed? Does he recognize you? Depressed patients may avoid eye contact.

The hand contact is useful. Some delirious or demented patients may not respond — they do not recognize the social gesture. This should alert you to the fact that all may not be well with the brain. Furthermore, the hand contact is of social significance for most of us. Frightened elderly patients may clutch, and maintain hand contact long after the formal handshake. Rarely, you may be surprised by the patient's unwillingness to let go; this may be a positive grasp reflex (a primitive reflex usually indicating damage to the frontal lobe of the brain, and common in demented patients). The hand contact is the first step to building up a rapport.

Giving your name and your purpose helps put the person at ease. It also helps you to assess short-term memory. You can ask the person subsequently 'Can you remember my name?' — if he cannot this may indicate cognitive impairment, but more usually suggests that he was not listening too carefully. It may be useful to write your name down for the person, with your contact address or phone number. This helps build up trust.

Ask the person 'What is your name?'. Be on the look-out for hearing impairment at this stage. The reply should give an idea about how the person wishes to be addressed. A first name, if given in response, should not be assumed to be the preferred form of address. For example, ask the patient, 'Would you like me to call you Mary, or do you prefer Mrs Jones?' By asking about forms of address you avoid calling a spinster Mrs, rather than Miss, and you also avoid being over-formal with those people who would rather be known by their first name.

POSITIONING, VISION AND HEARING

If you or your patient are uncomfortable you will not get very far. Make sure that the patient is in an appropriate position for what you plan to do. If you are simply going to talk to the patient, make sure he is sitting up, and preferably in a chair. If you are going to examine the legs, make sure the patient is in bed or on a couch. Get yourself a chair, and sit down so that you are not towering over the patient in an authoritarian way. It only takes a moment, and saves time later.

Remember that if you or the patient wants to go to the lavatory, the interview will be a tense business. Ask patients if they are comfortable, and check that they do not want to go to the lavatory. You may be the first person who has come near them and stopped long enough to ask since they came to the hospital.

Ask the patient if he usually wears glasses and ensure that the patient puts them on. If speech sounds slurred and the patient does not appear to have false teeth in place, ask where they are, and suggest they be put in. Ask about a hearing aid and make sure it is switched on. It is important in a hospital or nursing home to note the presence of such aids. Frequently they are 'lost' and a note in the case records stating that they were left at home is invaluable in finding them. Also, any regularly used aids should be obtained and used while the patient is in hospital.

Deafness is such a common problem that any situation where elderly people are seen regularly should have a communication aid. The simplest form of ear trumpet is often as effective as much more sophisticated electronic aids. Doctors should carry a small plastic trumpet in their 'black bags', and every ward in a hospital should have a supply. Shouting in the ear of a deaf patient is exhausting for everyone. Avoid doing it.

THE ENVIRONMENT

Talking at the bedside in a busy hospital ward is accepted practice in the UK. Provided the conversation is about general matters, and you are not too bothered whether the patient tells you the truth or not, go ahead and continue with the traditional approach. If you wish to talk about sensitive matters, or give the patient an opportunity to raise serious issues, do not try to do it behind the curtains in a shared room. This is not privacy, and it is only an institutionalized doctor who could possibly believe it is. It takes time to take a patient to the ward interview room, or to a quiet treatment room — but it is worth the time if you want to do the job properly. Your patients will notice the difference. A busy, noisy ward environment is exactly the wrong place to be talking about incontinence, testing for cognitive impairment, and exploring depressive symptoms and your patient's doubts and fears.

Furthermore, your pockets are never big enough to include the vision test board (Snellen chart), the auroscope and ophthalmoscope, the blood pressure machine, the rectal examination tray, the neurological examination kit, the tape measure, the goniometer, and so on. These should all be kept in one place, preferably a ward examination room.

If you do have to work in the main ward area, behind the curtains, do not forget that everyone else can hear what is going on. Furthermore, if you are called away, pull back the curtains so that your patient is not left in isolation.

GETTING THE STORY

Let the patient tell the story as he wishes, but help him with time sequence. It is useful to ask the patient: 'What happened to you today, why have you come into hospital?' This encourages the patient to focus on recent events. Inevitably, some patients will start: 'It all really started when I was gassed in the First World War.' Politeness dictates that you should listen to a little of the story. What the patient is saying to you is: 'I am a person who has been around, I've fought for my country, I am somebody.' You may use the story to collect information that you were planning to ask about later. For example, you might go on to ask about occupational history, about major life events besides the war, about past medical history. Although medical students are taught to start with the history of the presenting complaint, our patients are not taught this!

It is not worth spending time collecting information directly from the patient that can be more easily obtained from the case records, or family doctor's letter. Check important facts, but do not press the patient for dates of operations, or consultants' names. It is worth asking patients about their medication. Do they know the names of drugs, their purposes, and when they are meant to take them?

Interruptions. Try to avoid interrupting a patient's story if possible. Some patients give a rapid account of things, others are much slower. Try to adjust your pace to that of the patient.

Elderly patients have been around for a lot longer than younger patients, and have more to tell you. However, it is often necessary to interrupt and redirect the conversation. It is not impolite to do this, and you need to develop your own technique to avoid embarrassing the patient, or losing rapport. A comment to demonstrate you have been listening to what has just been said, followed by 'Can we just get back to the pain you were telling me about. Exactly where was it?', should help you get back on track.

Time. Doctors and nurses are busy people, they even walk quicker than most normal people! But do not fall into the trap of behaving like a 'busy person'. Your job is to talk to patients, and part of the skill is to make patients feel that they have your undivided attention. If you can, leave your bleep with the ward receptionist or with a colleague who can call you if a message is really urgent. Make sure you are not trying to do a 30-minute task if you have to be somewhere else in 10 minutes. Rather than do a rushed job, initially do a limited history or examination and come back later.

If you are called away in the middle of the interview, apologize and explain what is happening. Do not just run out of the room.

Embarrassing questions. Asking about incontinence, about sex life, about depressive symptoms can be embarrassing for both patient and doctor. It is even more difficult if you are not sensitive about how you ask the questions. Avoid asking direct questions like 'Are you ever incontinent?' Some patients may not understand the term 'incontinence', others may deny the symptom. A gentler and more effective question is: 'Do you ever have trouble holding your water?' It may be helpful to start a sensitive question like this: 'Some women find that sexual intercourse becomes quite painful after the menopause. Have you ever found that?'

It is best to keep sensitive questions until you have built up a rapport with a patient. Come back later. Start by showing that you respect the patient as a person. Admire a bedside photograph or Get Well card, or the patient's appearance. After the interview thank the patient for their clarity and helpfulness in giving a good history.

THE CONFUSED PATIENT

'Patient confused, no history available' speaks volumes about the training and attitudes of the medical profession. Confused patients deserve better. They are suffering from acute or chronic brain failure yet doctors seem inadequately trained to face up to the challenge of making a diagnosis and initiating management. Failure of almost any other organ system in the human body causes doctors to get excited and strive to find the underlying cause. Not so brain failure.

Many patients with major cognitive impairments (e.g. short-term memory loss, problems of recognition, language problems) are passed as normal by inexperienced (and sometimes experienced) professionals. In part this is because a patient needs a very small repertoire of social skills to maintain a facade of normality in the typical hospital ward, and even in front of his or her GP.

It is crucial to establish early on whether the patient is orientated in place, time and person. You also must decide whether the patient is alert. Mild degrees of clouding of consciousness are difficult to detect. The patient may appear to be 'not quite all there'.

ABBREVIATED MENTAL TEST (AMT)

- Age

- Time (to nearest hour)

- Address for recall

- Year

- Where do you live (town or road)?

- Recognition of two persons

- Date of birth (day and month)

- Year of start of First World War

- Name of present monarch

- Count backwards 20 to 1

- Don't forget to ask for the address!

Figure 18.2 Abbreviated mental test (AMT)

Most geriatricians now use a standard test of mental function (an example is shown in Fig. 18.2). Beware of announcing to the patient, and usually the rest of the ward, that you are about to ask her some 'silly questions'. By implication either you or the patient is silly to want to use such questions. Rather explain that you want to test your patient's memory, and ask him whether he minds you doing this. With experience it is possible to check most of the items in a mental test score by working them into your introductory talk with the patient. This is preferable to simply going through them like a shopping list. Remember that subtle impairment may not be detectable with a simple mental test score. You can try asking patients about current affairs, and for more information about their families.

Deafness and speech impairments, such as nominal dysphasia, can make patients *appear* very cognitively impaired, and depressed patients do not generally do well on mental test scores. On the other hand, confused patients can often reliably tell you about symptoms they are experiencing at the time; for example, do ask about pain and breathlessness.

ACTIVITIES OF DAILY LIVING (ADL)

Elderly people typically suffer with multiple pathology, some of which may be related to the reason for admission to hospital, or for consultation, some of which may not. A patient may give a symptom of chest pain suggesting a heart attack, prompting a detailed enquiry about cardiovascular and respiratory symptoms.

In young patients, a brief 'systems enquiry' concerning gastrointestinal, neurological and locomotor systems is all that is necessary to rule out significant (life-threatening) problems. In older patients this approach is not appropriate: a systems enquiry in an older patient can take almost forever, producing spurious symptoms. This is because elderly people may have so many symptoms, many of which are not relevant to the problem in hand. Some sort of screening is needed, and enquiry about activities of daily living provides a useful screen (see Fig. 18.3).

In general, patients who can dress, get about outdoors, are continent, can do their own housework and cooking, and manage their own pension, do not require much enquiry other than about their presenting problem. Such patients are the exception in usual practice with the old old and the oldest old.

If a daily living task cannot be carried out, then it is necessary to make a detailed enquiry focused on the reasons for this.

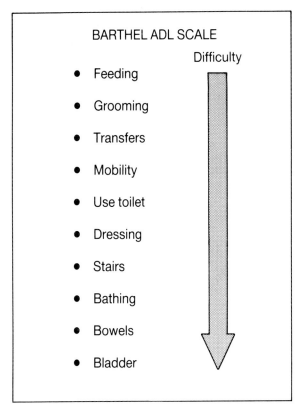

Figure 18.3 Barthel ADL scale

It is useful to obtain a 'pre-morbid' ADL, enabling you to describe what the patient is usually able to do before they became ill. This provides a rough goal for the outcome of treatment. A patient who was unable to get in and out of the bath, who could not dress, and who was incontinent prior to suffering a stroke or heart attack is not likely to get back to a trouble-free life. With younger patients we make the assumption that they were free from disability before the onset of an acute illness; with older people this assumption is seldom worth making.

A DRUG HISTORY

Old people are the pharmaceutical industry's greatest friend. They are prescribed more medication than any other age group.

Many patients, however, do not take all their prescribed medication. Check dates on tablet bottles and count the number of pills remaining as a rough guide to compliance. Everyone, young and old,

stashes medicines against some future catastrophe, so there are few medicine cabinets in the country that do not contain some out-of-date hypnotics, skin ointments and analgesics. Remember, too, that sharing of medication is commonplace as part of the self-help culture of elderly people — people swap stories about symptoms and try each other's drugs. Traditional treatment may also be used, and some people are naturally reluctant to divulge their secret remedies.

A TREATMENT HISTORY

- Current medication

- Previous hospital and family doctor medication

- Treatment from 'alternative' practitioners

- Self-medication

- Past bad experiences with medicines

- Other non-drug treatments

- Medicines kept in the home

Figure 18.4 A treatment history

Use Fig. 18.4 as a checklist when enquiring about current and past medications.

CORROBORATION OF THE EVIDENCE

None of us is a perfect witness of events, even if they concern us intimately. In medicine it is necessary to be critical of the history and check key points. (Most students are familiar with that sinking feeling when the consultant, having heard the student's history-taking, asks two or three questions of the patient that appear to totally contradict the main thrust of the history just elicited.) Patients change their story not because they are contrary, but because they become more astute to the importance of certain symptoms, they remember time relationships better, and sometimes it really is very difficult to be precise about a symptom.

The simplest method of corroboration is to go over the key symptoms with the patient after a few hours. However, it is essential to get whatever help you can from collateral sources of information. Obtain any old case notes from another hospital, because buried in them may be important information. Ring up the family doctor for clarification of points not covered in a referral letter. Most important of all, talk to a close relative or friend if at all possible. The telephone is a vital piece of equipment for history-taking with elderly patients. If you have not had to use it, ask yourself why not.

EXAMINATION

It is impossible to take a history and examine an elderly patient fully in under an hour. It is also unwise to try to spend an uninterrupted hour doing this. You will be exhausted and so will your patient. Your examination findings may well be inaccurate because of tiredness, so do not even try to do it all in one go (see Fig. 18.5). Take your history and then go away and write it down. You will inevitably have forgotten to ask for some vital piece of information, and you will almost always need to check important facts with case notes, the family doctor or a relative.

Come back to do your examination when you have thought through what it is you need to examine. Does the history suggest a neurological problem? Does the patient look Parkinsonian? Are you going to have to do a pelvic examination? Often it is worth doing a neurological examination as a separate exercise to achieve satisfactory cooperation.

Be gentle! Elderly skin bruises easily, and a rough hand does nothing to promote confidence that what will come later (e.g. taking blood, a rectal examination) will be done with care. Always explain what you intend to do, and help the patient into the appropriate position. Make sure your instructions are easy to understand.

Elderly people once possessed bodies as beautiful as your own, and they are only too aware of the effects

---

EXAMINATION OF A PATIENT

System	Don't forget!
General	Appearance, mood, skin Parkinson's, myxoedema anaemia, breasts, temperature, nutrition
CNS	Higher cortical tests, apraxia, agnosia, speech hemiparesis, wasting, vision, hearing
CVS / respiratory	Respiration rate, postural BP, scars
Abdominal	Bladder, PR, urine
Locomotor	Gait, transfers, feet, hips, knees
Aids / appliances	Stick, hearing aid spectacles, teeth

You can't do it all in one go!

Figure 18.5 Examination of a patient

---

of age on collagen, and of the difficulty of looking good with a wayward body. Do not aggravate this by a look of distaste as you examine a corpulent belly, or slide your stethoscope and fingers into severe intertrigo under a pendulous breast. You are not immune to the ageing process, and your turn will come!

Always praise a patient for their cooperation and performance. Do not do the examination in total silence, because this can suggest that you have discovered something terrible. Explain what you are doing as you go, and comment reassuringly on what you find.

Clothing. It sometimes seems that the principle of dressing elderly hospital patients in their own clothes is done simply to stop doctors getting on with examining them! It takes time to undress patients, but it is useful to use that time to observe your patients' abilities. Ask patients to remove clothes themselves. Consider whether the patient can reach her feet, can she manage her buttons, can she unhook her bra strap? Is her balance good, can she get on to the examination couch herself? These points may be of use in making the diagnosis, and any difficulty with undressing should be assessed by the occupational therapist.

Having got the patient undressed, be sure to keep him or her comfortable. Make use of a blanket to protect the patient's dignity, and never leave patients undressed while you get on with seeing another patient — it always takes longer than expected.

If you are planning to do a vaginal examination, or if the patient seems rather agitated, get a nurse to help you. Remember that nurses, too, are busy people, so try to make the experience rewarding for them. Explain what you are doing and why, and involve the patient in the conversation.

'EXTRAS' FOR THE ELDERLY

Elderly patients require the same examination as younger patients but there some extras that are often forgotten. Check visual acuity and hearing, the feet, and the patient's teeth — false or real. Check pressure areas (heels, hips, sacrum, shoulders, elbows) for signs of skin breakdown. A lying and standing (sitting will do) blood pressure is mandatory for all patients. Counting the respiratory rate is a more useful examination than listening to the chest. Most elderly people have noisy lung bases, but if the respiratory rate is not raised it is unlikely that there is an acute problem. Rectal examinations are a required part of a full examination, yet are often omitted in all age groups.

A common omission from a neurological examination is consideration of higher cortical function — the bits that make us human. The examination tends to focus on cranial nerves and spinal reflex arcs rather than testing language, perception and memory. Pencil-and-paper tests can be invaluable in providing a global measure of competence. A favourite test is to present a circle of about 10–15 cm diameter and ask the patient to fill in the numbers to make a clock face. This test will be abnormal (see, for example, Fig. 18.6) in patients who have visual impairments, who have difficulty carrying out purposeful actions (apraxia), who have perceptual problems, or who are cognitively impaired.

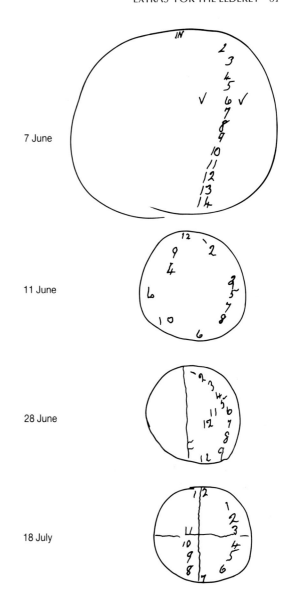

7 June

11 June

28 June

18 July

Figure 18.6 Clock face drawings: this patient showed some obvious improvement over the period

It is essential to examine every patient's walking — or gait pattern. Subtle evidence of hemiparesis may show up, as may poor balance, or the clutching 'furniture-cruising' gait of long-standing mobility problems. This also provides an objective check of at least one activity of daily living. Occasionally patients report that they are capable of carrying out activities when in reality they cannot.

Aids and appliances. Many patients have spectacles, hearing aids, dentures, walking sticks, wheelchairs, and many other aids. It is sensible to give them an examination too. A hearing aid that is not working is no use, so arrange to get it fixed. A walking stick with a worn ferrule may be dangerous on a wet pavement — change it. A wheelchair with flat tyres, or with worn brake pads, is both dangerous and an effort to use — get it overhauled. Elderly people's footwear is often ill-fitting and painful — get the physiotherapist, occupational therapist and surgical supplies staff to see what they can do.

Attention to detail. With elderly patients, more than with any other group it is attention to small, seemingly unimportant, details that makes the difference between success and failure. Because the details are not viewed as sufficiently important they are neglected, and so elderly patients fail to improve and get home. The satisfaction for health professionals in dealing with the details comes from the gratitude shown by patients who, for example have had chiropody for painful feet of years duration, or who can now hear after removal of impacted wax; and often simply from the fact that someone has *listened.*

EXPLANATION AND REASSURANCE

At the end of your history-taking and examination you should always explain what will happen next and when. Give a summary of what you think is the matter, and write down what you have told the patient. Check that the patient understands, by asking him or her to repeat the key points. Always ask patients if there is anything that has not been covered that they think you should know. Be sure to allow time for patients to ask you to clarify information.

Whether you have good or bad news for the patient at the end of the examination, be sure to reassure that everything will be dealt with properly, that the patient will be involved in deciding on how treatment will be organized, and leave the patient in no doubt that, no matter how serious the disease, you intend to do something helpful.

Key points

- Information obtained from the history is crucial in subsequent diagnosis and management. Even in a confused or dysphasic patient a history must be obtained by enquiry from relatives, friends, family doctors, nurses, wardens, and even the ambulance crew.
- Both you and the patient must be comfortable. A warm quiet room containing all the relevant equipment needed is essential.
- History-taking and examination takes a long time with a person who has lived a long time and has suffered many illnesses. Do not waste time establishing information that can be better obtained from old case records. Split the interview up to give both you and the patient a break.
- Use of a routine mental test examination, enquiry about performance of activities of daily living, and a careful drug history are essential.
- Elderly people take time to get undressed: observing any problems with undressing is an important part of the examination.
- Praise your patients for their help and cooperation, and reassure them as you carry out the examination. Explanations of what is the matter and what might be done are essential. Allow time for questions.
- Do not forget: visual acuity and hearing; feet and shoes; pressure areas; postural blood pressure; respiratory rate; higher cortical impairments (e.g. apraxias, agnosias); aids and appliances.

FURTHER READING

Bendall MJ. Examination of the elderly patient. In: Toghill P (ed.), *Examining Patients: An Introduction to Clinical Medicine.* Edward Arnold, London, 1990.

19 IMMOBILITY

- The cause
- The pattern of immobility
- Is the patient really immobile?
- What next?
- Mobilization

The immobile elderly patient is one of the classic and most common presentations. Every case requires careful history-taking to discover the underlying problems.

THE CAUSE

Ask the patient what has happened. Although obvious, this question is frequently omitted. A simple enquiry may lead to a direct lead (e.g. pain in the hip), an indirect lead (e.g. recurrent falls leading to fear of walking), or suggest important contributing factors (e.g. dementia or depression).

Separate cause from effect. It is all too easy to discover a diagnosis in an elderly patient and assume that this disease process is the cause of the patient's immobility. For example, a toxic confusional state may cause immobility, but immobility may be the cause of orthostatic pneumonia and dehydration.

Frequently it is not clear which way round events have occurred. The patient has several problems of which immobility is one. The management of the patient is not greatly influenced by sorting out the causal sequence, but the prognosis for recovery is largely determined by the underlying cause of the patient's immobility.

The last straw. Your patient may have been struggling along with several disabilities until a final event tipped the balance and pushed the patient into immobility. Often the last straw is a comparatively trivial problem (an inflamed bunion, or upper respiratory tract infection), or may be a 'social problem' such as a carer being taken ill, or a familiar home help going on holiday.

If the last straw that led to admission to hospital does seem minor to you, remember that this is simply an indication of the vulnerability of your patient. A trivial final cause of immobility does not make the fact of immobility any the less urgent a medical problem.

THE PATTERN OF IMMOBILITY

The crucial part of the history of immobility is the time frame. The graphs in Fig. 19.1 show several

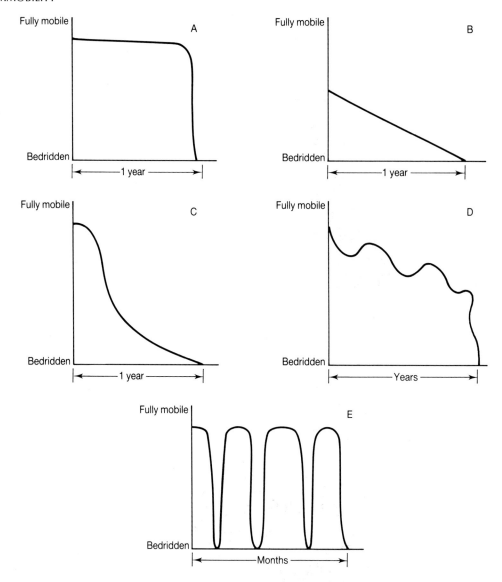

Figure 19.1 Five possible patterns of immobility

different possibilities. By the time you have finished taking the history you should be able to fit your patient into one of these patterns.

Patient A should be easy to sort out. Whatever caused the plunge into immobility occurred suddenly and recently. Diagnoses easily missed are stroke, impacted sub-capital hip fracture (often previously x-rayed in the Accident and Emergency department), toxic confusional state, and other acute medical diagnoses. Investigations will depend on your examination findings; but if these do not point to a clear

diagnosis, make sure you order a chest x-ray, ECG, cardiac enzymes, blood and urine cultures.

Patient B has a progressive disease process leading to steady deterioration in mobility. The disease may well have been diagnosed several years previously, so obtain the old medical records and go through the primary health care record in some detail. Old records may help chart the rate of decline, confirming its pattern. Parkinson's disease, myxoedema and osteoarthritis may show this sort of pattern.

Patient C is very difficult. Whatever caused the immobility happened a long time ago, and the picture is now clouded by complications of immobility. This patient will often have several diagnoses, none of which is the *cause* of the immobility. For example, the patient may have pneumonia, dehydration, pressure sores, muscle wasting, contracted joints, and a confusional state. The main task here is to decide on priorities for treatment (dehydration is usually top of the list), systematically ensuring that each problem is managed. As the patient's problems are solved, so it may become clearer what caused the original immobility.

Patient D has a stepwise decline, caused by a disease that has periods of exacerbation and of remission. Multiple sclerosis is the classic example, and can occur for the first time in old age. Chronic obstructive airways disease may produce this picture, as can recurrent heart attacks. Probably the commonest causes are recurrent minor strokes, and rheumatoid arthritis.

Patient E is interesting because of the rapid swings from full mobility to total immobility over a matter of days. Recurrent medical problems are a likely cause: heart failure, urinary tract infection, transient ischaemic attacks. Falls from whatever cause may lead to this sort of picture, with short periods of loss of confidence and immobility. If the periods of immobility are short (less than a day) it is worth considering Parkinsonian 'on–off' syndrome. Recurrent episodes of immobility often lead to recurrent hospital admissions. It is always worth making the effort of going through the notes, however thick they may be. It is all too tempting to label such patients as suffering from a behavioural or psychiatric problem, particularly when they get better without any apparent intervention. In such cases never overlook the possibility of alcohol abuse, other drug use (including prescribed medications), carbon monoxide poisoning from blocked flue pipes, and self-neglect due to depression or early dementia syndrome.

IS THE PATIENT REALLY IMMOBILE?

Having obtained an idea of the pattern of decline, and following a clinical examination, it is necessary to decide just how immobile your patient is. Within the bounds of common sense, you should get the patient standing and attempting a few steps.

This exercise may reveal the patient can walk, but is immobile because she is unable to get out of a bed or chair unaided. Alternatively, a confused patient may not have mentioned unbearable pain on standing or walking, which has prevented her from attempting to move.

A chair-shaped patient indicates a duration of immobility longer than a few days.

If the patient appears to have no concept of walking, suspect apraxia (inability to carry out a purposeful sequence of activity despite normal power and sensation) due to a stroke, dementia syndrome, or a confusional state.

Tentative steps, with clutching of helpers, may indicate loss of confidence following a fall.

If there is dramatic staggering to the nearest bed, chair or nurse followed by an Oscar-winning collapse, a behavioural cause is possible.

Sometimes a diagnostic gait pattern is found. Examples are: the broad-based gait of ataxia (poor balance); feet stuck to the floor (Parkinsonian syndrome); dragging of one leg (a stroke); waddling (weak proximal muscles — e.g. osteomalacia); or limp (joint disease, but also check feet).

Make sure that the patient can see. Blind people do not always tell the doctor!

WHAT NEXT?

There is seldom a shortage of diagnoses in an immobile patient; usually there are too many. A sensible strategy is to draw up a problem list, indicating possible causal relationships. The pattern and duration of immobility will give some indication of the chances of recovery. Each medical diagnosis will require treatment, although it is wise to set priorities and not attempt to treat everything at once. Rehydration and further use of the telephone are usually the first steps of management. A good problem list will ensure that you do not forget management of other, less pressing problems.

Immobility in elderly patients is almost always a multifactorial problem, so beware of coming down on a single diagnosis as the cause of immobility. 'Immobility due to Parkinson's disease' is more likely to be 'Immobility in a Parkinsonian patient because over-caring daughter tucked her up in bed when she had a cold. Unable to remobilize, now she has pneumonia'.

MOBILIZATION

The patient remains at risk of the complications of immobility even in hospital, so it is vital that a planned programme of mobilization starts as soon as possible. Do not confuse mobilization with moving the patient from bed to chair: very few elderly patients benefit from being nursed in a chair for long periods.

Some patients may find mobilization quite exhausting. It is always worth re-examining patients who are not progressing well. Often their poor exercise tolerance is due to undiagnosed heart failure, depression, muscle weakness, arthritis or pain. Appropriate treatment and advice usually allows continued, but slower, mobilization. Patients with dementia syndromes can be particularly difficult to mobilize, often they appear to be completely unwilling to do anything, and have virtually no ability to learn how to get back on their feet. In these cases it is important not to give up too soon, and a supportive team approach is vital. The physiotherapists cannot hope to mobilize such patients alone.

A small group of patients should not be mobilized rapidly: those with unstabilized fractures, vertebral collapse, bony secondaries, acutely inflamed joints, or joint effusions. In these cases the underlying disease process should be controlled first, and then mobilization started. For the majority, a progressive increase in activity, from lying to sitting on the edge of the bed, regaining postural reflexes, to taking a few steps with two helpers, to walking with a frame, to independent walking, should be attempted. It is not necessary to have a full diagnostic work-up before starting mobilization.

Key points

- Immobility is a classic presentation of disease, and may be caused by a wide range of different diseases. The aetiology is usually multifactorial, but often a single factor becomes 'the last straw'.
- The pattern of decline in mobility is fundamental to making a diagnosis and prognosis. Patterns are: sudden decline, progressive steady decline, sudden decline in distant past, stepwise decline, fluctuations.
- An essential part of the examination of all patients is to watch them stand up and walk, with assistance if necessary.
- Mobilization should begin as soon as any acute medical problem has been controlled, but should not wait until the whole team has completed their work-ups.

FURTHER READING

Andrews K. *Rehabilitation of the Older Adult.* Edward Arnold, London, 1987.

Bendall MJ, Bassey EJ, Pearson MB. Factors affecting walking speed of elderly people. *Age Ageing* 1989; **18**:327–32.

Imms RJ, Edholm OG. Studies of gait and mobility in the elderly. *Age Ageing* 1981; **10**:147–156.

Shephard RJ. *Physical Activity and Aging* (2nd edition) Croom Helm, London, 1987.

20 FALLS

- Causes
- Key questions to ask
- Psychological consequences of falls

Falls are common in old age, and are more common amongst women than men. The reported prevalence of falls over a period of a year is approximately 30 per cent, although prospective studies have given lower rates, suggesting that elderly people tend to overestimate their experience of falls when asked to recall past events.

Table 20.1 Physiological ageing changes

Reduced muscle strength
Slower psychomotor responses
Increased body sway
Poorer proprioception
Slower visual accommodation reflexes

As people age various physiological changes take place that increase their risk of falling (see Table 20.1). So-called accidental falls are often caused by a failure to respond quickly enough to change in the body's centre of gravity. Poorer proprioception is a factor, coupled with the need to use vision much more than at younger ages to correct and maintain balance.

Clearly it is sensible practice to make the home environment as safe as possible by removing loose mats and stair carpets, ensuring that lights are left on in dark hallways, fixing stair rails that go down beyond the last step, replacing wall sockets to waist height to avoid bending down, and re-siting kitchen cabinets and shelves at a height where things can be reached easily. However, many elderly people may view such alterations with little enthusiasm, so it is as well to consider such changes as part of a pre-retirement plan when behaviour may be easier to change.

CAUSES

Falls range from minor, trivial trips with no lasting consequences to major, life-threatening events. The underlying pathologies that cause falls are numerous. The aim of history taking and examination of a person seen because of falls is to attempt to diagnose the underlying pathological processes shown in Table 20.2. The physiological changes of ageing may well be superimposed on disease processes, making it a difficult task to sort out the underlying cause.

Premonitory falls occur in the run-up to a serious illness, and it is common for an elderly patient to have presented with a fall to an Accident and Emergency department the day before admission with pneumonia. Often careful assessment at the time of a premonitory fall will reveal signs of underlying acute illness. Casual assessment will not!

The more medications a patient takes the greater the risk of falling. This may be because of the drugs themselves, but is more likely a marker of serious underlying diseases. However, drugs that cause low blood pressure, particularly on standing up (postural hypotension), may cause falls. The most notorious are diuretics and antidepressants.

Table 20.2 The causes of falls

Premonitory falls
Forerunner of acute, usually infectious, illness

Prescribed medications
Multiple drugs
Psychotropic drugs
Diuretics
Antihypertensives
L-dopa

Neurological disease
Stroke
Transient ischaemic attack
Parkinson's disease
Cerebellar disease
Spinal cord degeneration
Epilepsy

Circulatory system diseases
Silent myocardial infarction
Vasovagal attack (faints, micturition syncope)
Dysrhythmias
Postural hypotension
Vertebrobasilar syndrome
Carotid sinus sensitivity

Musculo-skeletal disease
Generalized muscle weakness
Wasting secondary to arthritis
Unstable knee joint
Proximal myopathy

Miscellaneous
Drop attacks
Hypoglycaemia
Electrolyte imbalance
Pain (e.g. feet)
Abuse
Labyrinthitis
Cervical spondylosis
Alcohol
Environmental hazards
Poor vision

Neurological diseases are commonly associated with falls, and may be quite subtle and difficult to detect. Mild strokes are frequently not detected by a superficial examination. Parkinson's disease may not be associated with a tremor and can often be mistaken for 'ageing'. Although cerebellar disease is quite rare it often leads to a very unsteady, drunken gait, since the cerebellum is responsible for coordination and balance. Causes of cerebellar disease are strokes, myxoedema, alcoholism, and degeneration associated with cancers (especially of bronchus and breast).

The spinal cord carries both motor nerve fibres (pyramidal tracts) and position sensory fibres (posterior columns) to the brain. Vitamin B_{12} deficiency (pernicious anaemia) and neurosyphilis (tabes dorsalis) can both affect the spinal cord, and lead to a degeneration of both types of nerve fibre. Epilepsy is often due to a previous stroke in elderly people, although brain tumours may also cause epilepsy. An epileptic attack will lead to a fall, and without a witness to the attack this can be difficult to diagnose.

Circulatory system diseases are common. 'Silent' myocardial infarction (i.e. without characteristic chest pain) may present with a fall because of reduced cardiac output and low blood pressure, and associated heart failure. Vasovagal attacks (faints) can also occur in elderly people and may be precipitated by straining — for example on micturition. Dysrhythmias, often due to ischaemic heart disease, may lead to an abnormally slow heart rate or a very rapid heart rate. In both cases, cardiac output is reduced and a fall may result. Postural hypotension of up to 40 mmHg between lying and standing systolic blood pressure occurs in up to 5 per cent of elderly people, for no apparent reason. Such patients may feel extremely light-headed and dizzy on standing and are therefore at risk of falling. In many cases an underlying cause is found: drugs, myocardial infarction, dehydration, or acute blood loss from a bleeding peptic ulcer. Vertebrobasilar syndrome is probably over-diagnosed, and is thought to be due to interruption of the blood supply to the brainstem on upward or sideways movement of the head associated with cervical spondylosis. In true cases, associated symptoms of tinnitus, double vision and vertigo are found.

Musculoskeletal diseases are usually obvious, and may be due to general effects of widespread cancer, or local effects of arthritis. Osteoarthritis of the knee joints may lead to instability of the joint and the sensation of the joint 'giving' and may precipitate a fall. Less often seen is a proximal myopathy of the limb girdle muscles (shoulders or pelvis) which leads to difficulties getting out of a chair and climbing stairs. Osteomalacia sometimes causes this problem and improves with treatment with vitamin D and calcium.

Miscellaneous causes of falls are many, but drop attacks deserve special mention. The patient is usually walking outdoors, and in previously good health. Without any warning, the legs give way and the patient is unable to get up. The legs feel useless, but after a variable time (up to several hours) the use comes back into the legs and the patient is able to walk again. The underlying cause of drop attacks remains unkown.

Occasionally it is necessary to pose the question 'Did the patient fall, or was she pushed?' Elder abuse is increasingly recognized as a cause of trauma in frail elderly people.

The inner ear contains sensitive mechanisms for maintenance of balance, and acute viral labyrinthitis will lead to severe vertigo and nausea. The presentation is usually so acute and the symptoms severe, that diagnosis is not difficult. Lesser degrees of chronic dizziness are very common in elderly people and are frequently attributed to cervical spondylosis. However, x-ray changes in the cervical spine are so common that it is difficult to be certain that this is really the cause of the symptoms, and it is seldom the cause of recurrent falls.

Too much alcohol is a common cause of falling over at any age. It has to be remembered that some elderly people are likely to over-indulge in drinking; this, together with their poorer physiological mechanisms for maintaining balance, means that they are more likely to fall over after a relatively modest amount of alcohol.

KEY QUESTIONS TO ASK

It should be obvious that even a single fall should lead to a detailed history and examination. Witnesses should be questioned too; often this is not done, and opportunities for early diagnosis and treatment are missed. The family doctor and Accident and Emergency department staff are likely to be the first doctors to assess such patients, and need to give time, sympathy, and a systematic approach. Often referral to the Department of Health Care of the Elderly will be needed for diagnosis and treatment.

Is the patient in good health?

A fall in a patient who is suffering with a chronic disability should lead to a different line of enquiry. Many falls occur in the course of daily living (for example, transferring from bed to chair, or in the bathroom) in patients with previous strokes, Parkinson's disease, and arthritis. It is essential to make a careful enquiry about medication, and any recent changes.

In a patient who was previously well, a search must be made for new acute illness. If none is present, then the fall may be 'accidental' and due to ageing physiology, or due to environmental factors (poor lighting, loose mats).

Has the patient had previous falls?

Unless a fall leads to a severe consequence, such as a fracture, patients often to do not seek any medical attention. It is often only after recurrent or bad falls that help is sought. Recall of the pattern of previous falls can be helpful, in particular their frequency, relationship with posture, time of day, any residual symptoms following the fall, and any avoiding steps taken by the patient.

What was the patient doing at the time?

Falls that occur on changing posture, particularly lying to standing, suggest postural hypotension, vertebrobasilar insufficiency, or accidents. Coexisting diseases may lead to falls on transfers (see above).

Did the patient trip?

A trip may occur simply as the result of poor postural reflexes associated with ageing, but may be aggravated by poor vision. Sometimes bifocal glasses can give a distorted view, leading to an accidental fall. Outdoor falls may be due to uneven pavements, or being pushed by other people. Frequently, patients admit that they were trying to do two things at once (for example, boiling some soup when the doorbell rang) and in a moment of confusion over which task to attend to, a fall occurred.

Did the patient get any warning?

The absence of any warning implies a sudden event, usually of a neurological or circulatory nature. However, prior to an epileptic fit patients may feel peculiar, and can feel dizzy with the onset of any cause of a reduced cardiac output.

Is the patient able to walk normally?

Perhaps the single most useful investigation of elderly fallers is to watch them walking, as the signs of diseases that frequently cause falls may be ruled out: Parkinson's disease, stroke, arthritis, muscle weakness, neuropathy, cerebellar disease.

If the patient has a normal gait, it is necessary to rule out the transient causes of instability: epilepsy, dysrhythmias, postural hypotension, effects of drugs and alcohol, myocardial infarction, hypoglycaemia, transient ischaemic attacks.

PSYCHOLOGICAL CONSEQUENCES OF FALLS

A fall is a tremendous psychological blow to many elderly people. It reminds them of their increasing frailty, and may lead to dramatic loss of confidence, particularly walking outdoors. This in turn may lead to becoming housebound, and a reduction in social contacts, and depression. Many patients require protracted rehabilitation, with practice in their own homes and nearby shops to restore confidence. A medically trivial fall may have far-reaching effects on the individual.

Key points

- Falls are extremely common, with up to a third of people having a fall in the course of a year.
- Physiological ageing changes make older people more vulnerable to falls, but a search must be made for underlying diseases.
- Important points in the history are: is the patient in good health; has the patient had previous falls; what was the patient doing at the time; did the patient trip; was there any warning?
- The single most useful part of the examination is to watch the patient walking. A postural blood pressure reading is essential.

FURTHER READING

Blake AJ, Morgan K, Bendall MJ, *et al.* Falls in elderly people at home: prevalence and associated factors. *Age Ageing* 1988; **17**:365–372.

Campbell AJ, Spears GFS, Brown JS, Busby WJ, Borrie MJ. Circumstances and consequences of falls experienced by a community population 70 years and over during a prospective study. *Age Ageing* 1990; **19**:136–141.

Tinetti ME. Falls. In: Cassel CK, Riesenberg DR, Sorensen LB, Walsh JR (eds), *Geriatric Medicine*, 2nd edn. Springer-Verlag, London, 1990.

21 CONFUSION

- Acute confusion
- Chronic confusion (dementia)
- Alzheimer's disease
- Multi-infarct dementia
- Laboratory investigation
- Management

A confusional state is best described as being either acute or chronic.

ACUTE CONFUSION

Acute confusion (delirium) is one of the most common forms of organic brain syndrome with both physical and mental abnormalities needing urgent assessment. The clinical features are listed in Table 21.1. It is relatively uncommon in young people as their confusion threshold is high, although conditions such as malaria and severe pneumonia may cause confusion. The threshold for confusion is much lower in older people and it may be the presenting feature of such conditions as myocardial infarction, pneumonia or urinary tract infection. Failure to recognize it and hence to diagnose and treat the underlying condition can have fatal consequences for the patient. This is most likely to occur in patients already suffering from a chronic confusional state whose acute exacerbation is misinterpreted as simply a worsening of the 'dementia'. Failure to assess a person's level of cognitive functioning on admission and to monitor it periodically during hospitalization can also result in a missed diagnosis of acute confusional state. 'Acute' can mean an onset ranging from a few minutes through hours and days up to three months.

Table 21.1 Clinical features of acute confusion (delirium)

Clouding of consciousness
Disorientation in time and place
Onset usually over hours and days (fluctuating course)
Poor short term memory
Hallucinations or misinterpretations
Altered activity levels (agitated, restless and wandering or drowsy and lethargic)
Evidence of the disease process causing the confusion with physical signs — tachycardia, sweating, etc.
Speech abnormalities (mumbling, rambling).

There are major groups of causes of acute confusion (Table 21.2), though it is common to find multiple causes.

Prodromal features such as restlessness, hypersensitivity to visual and auditory stimuli, nocturnal insomnia and daytime sleepiness may all be found.

The factors shown in Table 21.3 are thought to predispose to acute confusion.

Table 21.2 Major causes of acute confusion

Neurological conditions: Head injury, stroke (especially small cortical lesions without focal neurological signs), epilepsy.

Systemic conditions: Infections, hypoxia/hypercarbia, uraemia, hypo/hyperglycaemia, hypo/hyperthermia, heart failure, myocardial infarction, pulmonary emboli, acid–base disturbance, after a 'fall'

Drugs: Side-effect of prescribed medication (anticholinergics, hypnotics/sedatives/tranquillizers, antidepressants, analgesics, L-dopa preparations) Overdose or withdrawal (alcohol, hypnotics)

Environmental changes: A move to new surroundings, e.g. admission to an institution (translocation effect) 'Sundowner' syndrome (increased agitation/confusion in people with chronic confusion in the evening)

Table 21.3 Factors that predispose to acute confusion

Ageing process (decreased threshold)
Impairment of vision and hearing
Presence of chronic physical and chronic brain disease
Age-related changes in drug effects

Early diagnosis is important because most patients can recover with appropriate treatment. However advanced age and longer duration of illness worsen the prognosis and mortality rates range up to 30 per cent. The differential diagnoses include acute on chronic confusion, chronic state (e.g. the dementias) and acute functional psychosis (pseudodelirium).

Treatment

Specific. This is directed at the underlying pathology and may involve treating acute illnesses such as infections or myocardial infarction using appropriate drugs and other help (e.g. nursing care, physiotherapy).

Supportive. Initially the patient may need intensive nursing care, and this is best carried out in a well-lit single room with the minimum of disturbance. Avoid frequent changes of staff, loud noises, and other disruptions. Cot-sides should not be used. If the person is severely agitated, and whilst waiting for treatments to work, the mattress can be placed on the floor (after explaining to carers) to avoid serious injury. Severely ill patients may need intravenous therapy. Less ill but still restless patients may prefer to be up in a chair.

Once a diagnosis has been made and a plan of treatment organized it is best if at all possible to let the specific medication work and the confusional state settle. This may require a dedicated nurse to encourage fluids, reassure, monitor vital signs and help prevent restlessness. However, some patients are very agitated and occasionally violent or are a danger to themselves by being so unsteady that some calming medication is necessary. Haloperidol is an excellent drug for this purpose, having flexibility of administration and dosage. The smallest effective dose should be used; the aim is *not* to render a difficult patient unconscious only to wake up for someone else to deal with. Other suitable agents are thioridazine and chlormethiazole. Chlorpromazine should be avoided. The drugs should only be given for a short time and withdrawn as soon as the organic cause of the confusional state responds to treatment.

An assessment of mental state is not complete without a *mental test score*. This appraisal of short- and long-term memory, orientation and numeracy skills can be performed using a simple plan like that in Fig. 18.2 in Chapter 18, or more elaborate forms such as the mini-mental state examination. Highly complex tests (some using user-friendly computers) are available and advice can be obtained from a clinical psychologist for both acute and chronic confusional states.

The mental test score is most valuable when used on the same patient over a period of time. A low initial score becomes more relevant if an underlying diagnosis of dementia is suspected and it does not improve after treatment of any acute problems. A score that rapidly improves over a few days obviously helps rule out a chronic 'dementing' illness.

CHRONIC CONFUSION (DEMENTIA)

Chronic confusional states must have been present for at least three months to be labelled as such. There is usually loss of function in multiple areas (e.g. intellectual function, memory, language). There are, however, *reversible* causes, so appropriate diagnosis and treatment may produce improvement. Chronic confusional states become increasingly common in old age (10 per cent above age 65, 20 per cent above age 80) but are obviously not a component of normal ageing. Regardless of age a search for the cause is warranted in most cases (see Table 21.4).

The differential diagnoses include acute confusional states, benign (senile) forgetfulness, amnestic syndromes, and depression (pseudodementia).

Table 21.4 Major causes of chronic confusion

Reversible causes (about 20 per cent of cases)
Drugs (e.g. long-acting tranquillizers)
Endocrine disorders (e.g. hypothyroidism)
Systemic illness
Vitamin deficiencies (e.g. B 12, thiamine)
Under-nutrition
Intracranial masses (benign and resectable) (e.g. meningioma)
CNS infections (e.g. syphilis)
Normal pressure hydrocephalus (see Fig. 21.1)
Depression
Alcohol

Irreversible causes
Alzheimer's disease
Pick's disease
Multi-infarct dementia
CNS malignancy
Creutzfeldt–Jacob disease
Huntington's disease
Parkinson's disease
Postinfective brain damage
AIDS 'dementia'
Post-traumatic/anoxic brain damage

Figure 21.1 A rare cause of confusion: normal pressure hydrocephalus shown on a CT scan

Acute confusional states (or acute on chronic) should be picked up by the presence of specific features (clouding of consciousness, evidence of the disease process with physical signs, etc.). Benign (senile) forgetfulness involves a minor degree of forgetfulness especially for recent memory (sufferers are forever losing keys, spectacles, etc.). It was portrayed to perfection by Margaret Rutherford in the film *The VIPs*. It is not progressive. The amnestic syndromes include alcohol abuse (Korsakoff's syndrome secondary to thiamine deficiency), trauma (including the repeated head trauma of boxers — dementia pugilistica), hypoxia and stroke. Transient global amnesia is a condition of short-lived amnesia (usually hours) secondary to either migraine or cerebral microemboli. Depression can be difficult to distinguish from a primary chronic confusional state and in some cases a psychiatric opinion should be sought. A diagnosis of depression may be helped by the findings of a more rapid onset and progression of symptoms and a depressed mood. Attention and concentration as well as learning abilities are often intact.

The multiple cognitive 'losses' are of sufficient severity to interfere with social and occupational functioning. The deficits being multifaceted involve memory, judgement, abstract thought and a variety of higher cortical functions. Changes in personality and behaviour also occur and these may cause the greatest distress to carers.

Memory impairment is the most prominent symptom, especially recent memory. In mild cases there is forgetfulness in daily life and the need for repetition to facilitate remembering. In severe cases long-term memory is also affected. Impairment of abstract thinking can be assessed by testing the ability to interpret proverbs. Language (a higher cortical function) is often impaired; it may become vague, stereotyped, imprecise or aphasic. Dyspraxia (the inability to perform common tasks such as dressing or walking) also occurs. Judgement becomes impaired and personality changes, including the accentuation of pre-existing traits (e.g. aggression, paranoia), are common. Some people retain a degree of insight and not unnaturally become depressed; others suffer from anxiety. In advanced cases they may have delusions or hallucinations.

The above description applies mainly to the largest group of non-reversible causes of chronic confusion — the dementing syndromes.

The two most common causes of dementia are Alzheimer's disease and multi-infarct dementia.

Alzheimer's disease is seen more frequently in clinical practice but a positive diagnosis of either of the two conditions requires careful assessment. Post mortem histological studies of brain tissue, however, shows a great deal of overlap between the two conditions.

ALZHEIMER'S DISEASE

Alzheimer's disease was named by Alois Alzheimer in 1907. He described senile plaques and neurofibrillary tangles in the brain sections of a 57-year-old woman who died of 'dementia'. His name became attached to this pre-senile form although it is very rare. The similar condition in the elderly was termed senile dementia of the Alzheimer type (SDAT). Now all cases are termed Alzheimer's disease (AD).

AD is a clinical diagnosis made by excluding other disorders. A definitive diagnosis can only be made by biopsy (not usually feasible) or at autopsy. The characteristic histopathological changes are neurofibrillary tangles, neuritic plaques and amyloid angiopathy especially in the hippocampus, temporal-parietal-occipital junction and in the nucleus basalis of Meynert. Other findings include diffuse cortical atrophy, diminished brain weight, gliosis and granulovacuolar degeneration. These findings are not pathognomonic for they occur in other disease processes and in *normal ageing*, the difference being quantitative, and in the location of the changes. Investigations are usually normal, although a CT brain scan may show some non-specific cortical atrophy.

The discovery of a cholinergic deficiency in AD was a major advance in research. The replacement of neurochemical transmitters is a fundamental research area that may produce new treatments in the future.

Finding a 'cause' for Alzheimer's disease revolves around three other research topics: the role of aluminium; a viral aetiology; and the role of genetics. Aluminium is the world's most abundant metal, being present in all food chains and the water supply. It forms the core of the neuritic plaque found in the disease. In parts of the world where the element is present in high levels there appears to be a higher incidence of neurological disorders (in some places clinical combinations of AD, Parkinson's disease and multiple sclerosis). Aluminium is certainly neurotoxic as evidenced by the damage caused to renal dialysis patients when dialysis fluid was originally found to contain high aluminium levels.

There is currently no evidence to favour a viral/slow virus aetiology for AD, although it is well recognized that transmissible agents (probably smaller than viruses) are responsible for at least two dementia syndromes — Kuru in Papua New Guinea, and Creutzfeld–Jacob disease. The intense interest in the species transmission of Bovine spongiform encephalitis (BSE or 'Mad Cow' disease) has revived speculation concerning transmissable 'dementing' agents.

Down's syndrome may help provide a genetic 'marker' for the disease. Down's patients develop histopathological changes similar to AD at an early age. The genetic defect is known in Down's syndrome, so presumably the 'code' for the brain damage is present in this segment and when accurately located could be isolated, possibly providing a marker to susceptibility. It is now known that the precursor protein for amyloid is coded for by a gene on the long arm of the chromosome 21 and another gene in this location governs some cases of the familial form of AD that affects younger people.

MULTI-INFARCT DEMENTIA

Multi-infarct dementia results when patients have sustained recurrent cortical or subcortical strokes.

Table 21.5 Investigations for chronic confusion

Necessary
Blood count and film
ESR
Kidney and liver function
Glucose
Calcium and phosphate
Thyroid function
Vitamin B_{12} and red cell folate
Syphilis serology
Chest x-ray
ECG
CT brain scan

In selected cases
EEG
HIV screen
Lumbar puncture
Blood cultures
Blood gases
Toxicity screen

Most of the strokes are too small to cause permanent damage or even residual focal neurological deficits. The clinical criteria for vascular dementia includes the presence of a dementia with a stepwise deteriorating course, a patchy or uneven distribution of cognitive deficits, and focal neurological signs. Other characteristic features include the presence of hypertension, signs of atherosclerotic disease elsewhere, emotional lability, pseudobulbar palsy, dysarthria and transient depression. The Hachinski score gives 'marks' for each of the above and a score over 4 is consistent with multi-infarct dementia.

LABORATORY INVESTIGATIONS

The use of investigations in chronic confusional states is aimed at identifying potentially reversible causes. At the same time one must not subject vulnerable patients to unpleasant tests or waste resources. Table 21.5 lists investigations that should be considered in patients with a relatively short history who are otherwise well.

MANAGEMENT

This section can only give the briefest outline to a subject area that is one of the most difficult in all medicine. The stress, anxiety and concern of relatives and carers cannot be overestimated. One fundamental aim is to try to optimize the patient's function. Underlying medical disease should be treated with the avoidance of medication with CNS side-effects. The patient's environment can be assessed and alterations suggested which encourage physical and mental activity. Memory aids should be used and good nutrition encouraged. New medical complications need to be quickly identified and treated. Once the diagnosis is made it should be explained fully to carers, and advice given on sources of future help, including the Alzheimer's Disease Society. Early preparation for any changes in residence should be made and problems such as wandering, behaviour disorders, depression, agitation or aggressiveness need to be discussed, and where necessary, involve a local psychiatrist.

Help is usually multidisciplinary and should as far as possible occur in the patient's home. There should be regular reassessment of function and medical checks. Family/carers (and where possible the patient) should be kept informed. Some may want to know the nature of the disease, the extent of impairment and prognosis. Links should be made early with social services and voluntary organizations, since each district provides different and sometimes unique services (night sitters, legal and financial counselling, relative support groups).

The counselling aspect is particularly important with a view to identifying and resolving family conflict, handling anger and guilt, helping with decisions over respite or institutional care, legal and indeed ethical issues.

Key points

- A confusional state is best described as being acute or chronic.
- Acute confusion (delirium) has both physical and mental abnormalities needing urgent assessment.
- Clouding of consciousness is an important feature of acute confusion (others include disorientation, poor short-term memory, hallucinations and evidence of a disease process).
- Acute confusion may be the presenting feature of almost any medical condition in an elderly person.
- Common causes of acute confusion include stroke, infections and medication.
- Treatment is specifically directed at the underlying pathology. Supportive measures include a well-lit room and the minimum of disruption.
- Assessment of the mental state is essential in all cases of confusion.
- The mental test score is most valuable when used on the same patient over a period of time.
- Twenty per cent of cases of chronic confusion have a potentially reversible cause.
- Reversible causes of chronic confusion include drugs, endocrine abnormalities and depression.
- Alzheimer's disease and multi-infarct dementia are two of the most common dementia syndromes.
- Research in Alzheimer's disease involves cholinergic pathways, replacement therapy as well as the role of aluminium, viruses and genetic markers.
- In most cases patients with chronic confusional states require investigation.

FURTHER READING

Arie T. Confusion in old age. *Age Ageing* 1978; **7** (Suppl):72–76.

Bennett GCJ. *Alzheimer's Disease and Other Confusional States.* Macdonald Optima, London, 1989.

Hachinski VC. Multi-infarct dementia: a cause of mental deterioration in the elderly. *Lancet* 1974; **ii**:207–209.

Small GW, Jarvik LF. The dementia syndrome. *Lancet* 1982; **ii**:1443–1446.

22 INCONTINENCE

- Definition
- Acceptable places
- Getting there
- History and examination
- Urinary incontinence
- Faecal incontinence

As babies our bladders and bowels function involuntarily and automatically. In early childhood we are trained to identify acceptable places and control excretion by the discipline of praise (keeping dry and not wetting the bed). Once control has been achieved any failure causes embarrassment which continues to occur at any age. To avoid this only 'acceptable' voiding is allowed, so an individual must be able to identify an acceptable place and get there safely. Advancing age and increasing disability can lower the threshold for control but incontinence is not an inevitable outcome of ageing.

DEFINITION

Incontinence is an involuntary loss of urine or faeces in an inappropriate place. This implies that there were no physical or psychological barriers preventing access to an acceptable place but despite this one excreted inappropriately. This necessitates a thorough investigation as many causes of involuntary loss

of control are amenable to medical and surgical management.

ACCEPTABLE PLACES

These are dependent upon a host of factors such as age, sex, social class, society, nationality, and present circumstances. The driver of a hansom cab is allowed by law to urinate against the rear offside wheel of his cab. This law has never been repealed, but putting it to the test would probably result in an arrest for obscene behaviour in a public place. Peasant farmers squat down in fields around the world, but Oxford Street (which was once a field) is certainly not now acceptable, society here has decreed the use of private lavatories or public conveniences. Most people have no problem in identifying acceptable places. Difficulties arise, however, when one is unaware of the location. This can happen to anyone in a strange town or building and is a plight experienced by people with dementia; they know they should get to an acceptable place but they cannot find it. If directed, continence results, if not the nearest suitable alternative (bin or sink) is used rather than be wet. There is no difference in behaviour between the demented patient and someone unable to find a toilet who urinates in the bushes or up against a wall.

In hospitals the lack of suitable toilets is a common cause of loss of continence. Patients may be aware of the need to go, of where to go and of acceptable alternatives (commodes) but are unable to get to them in time. Some patients are placed on incontinence pads in bed, psychologically inviting loss of control. The necessity to get up at night to urinate increases with advancing age. High beds, night sedatives, cot-sides and shortage of help combine to prevent patients from getting to the toilet. It is essential that commodes and toilets be near the beds and chairs of elderly patients.

GETTING THERE

Psychological barriers

The indignity of being inadequately clothed (split-back nightdresses, trouser bottoms that fall down) leads to many people being incontinent rather than shame themselves crossing a semi-public ward area.

Loss of mobility

This is the commonest cause of difficulty both in the community and in institutions. Most public conveniences were designed for the physically able. There are few with disabled access and disabled facilities. People taking diuretics or those with bladder or bowel control difficulties often have to plan routes on the basis of available toilet facilities; more commonly they become housebound. There is no need for architects and town planners to experience being old; a test dose of a fast-acting diuretic taken in the middle of a shopping precinct should concentrate the mind!

Location of toilet

An outside toilet requires that to be continent one must get outside (whatever the weather) or use another receptacle. Toilets upstairs depend on good physical mobility. Thus many elderly people who are ill at home have been 'incontinent' before they enter hospital, their illness preventing them from reaching the toilet. The loss of control is due to illness and associated immobility, not their age. A bedside com-mode may have enabled them to remain continent. How they are treated in hospital will influence whether incontinence becomes an established pattern or not.

Ward toilets

The majority of hospital wards have too few toilets, often providing only two for 20–30 people. If we really expected people to be continent we would provide (as in hotels) a lavatory for each patient next to the bed. Most patients have to walk long distances and then wait. Toilet doors are often heavy and the space may not permit a wheelchair or walking frame. Unless specifically designed the seat will be too low, with no hand rails and toilet paper on a roll. Try going to the toilet using only one hand, balancing on one leg and get a few pieces of paper off the roll at a time (this is often the situation stroke patients find themselves in).

Bad design

Many hospitals are still equipped with old-fashioned high beds so that nearly all elderly patients need assistance to get in and out. If someone does try to get out unaided they either fall or sides are put up. If the bed is adjustable and set correctly most patients can get out unaided and cot-sides are certainly unnecessary.

Use of bed pans

The gymnastic prowess necessary to straddle a bed pan and maintain balance and position on it is difficult and exhausting for most elderly patients. The sheer act becomes one of dread and putting off its use can lead to retention and constipation with later faecal incontinence due to overflow (spurious diarrhoea). A bedside commode is easier to use.

Chairs

The correct chair is one that a person can get out of easily. Properly dressed (with underclothes), sitting in a chair of the correct height with a walking frame nearby, the majority of elderly patients can get to the toilet independently. They cannot do this if the chair is too high or too low, if they are trapped by a fixed table or if they feel inadequately dressed or cannot reach their walking frame.

HISTORY AND EXAMINATION

A full clinical history with careful attention to the history of bladder and bowel function prior to the present illness (from both patient and relatives) will help to differentiate between loss of ability to control excretion and failure to identify or get to an acceptable place. Clinical examination, including a rectal and a vaginal examination, and culture of a mid-stream specimen of urine are all essential (and will often give a good indication as to the cause of the problem).

An incontinence chart kept for a few days only (it is a very nurse-intensive process) may give a recognizable pattern of urine (and/or faecal) incontinence (e.g. morning incontinence associated with fast-acting diuretics). The specialist help of a continence adviser may be needed.

URINE

Causes

The common causes of urinary incontinence are listed in Table 22.1 and the mechanisms in Table 22.2.

Table 22.1 Common causes of urinary incontinence

Urinary tract infection
Stress incontinence
Detrusor instability (unstable bladder)
Retention with overflow
Prostatism
Uninhibited neurogenic bladder
Reflect neurogenic bladder
Atonic neurogenic bladder
Others
   Uterine prolapse
   Cystocoele
   Atrophic vaginitis

Table 22.2 Mechanisms of urinary incontinence

Involuntary detrusor contractions
Loss of normal elasticity of bladder wall
Incompetence of bladder neck and distal sphincter
   mechanisms
Loss of higher CNS control of micturition function
Abnormalities of bladder sensation

Infection

Urinary tract infections are common — there is a 20 per cent incidence in people over 65 years (compared with 3.2 per cent in the age group 45–65 years). They are potentially very serious.

Less efficient bladder emptying (especially if there is any degree of bladder neck obstruction) may predispose to an increased frequency of infection. Women wiping bowel organisms forwards to the urethral area can also precipitate infection. Other pathologies in the urinary tract presenting with infection (e.g. bladder tumours, stones) should be considered. The classic history of frequency and dysuria is often absent. A urinary tract infection may present as an acute confusional state or a series of falls, and because it is so common should always be ruled out by appropriate testing, including dipstix tests done on the ward.

Stress incontinence

In this condition there is bladder neck incompetence; the distal urethral mechanism is unable to cope with the intra-abdominal pressure rise that occurs on coughing and laughing. It is extremely common in women and has been related to the 'damage' that occurs to the pelvic musculature during childbirth. In addition the post-menopausal changes (due to the lack of oestrogen) give rise to atrophic change affecting the muscular sphincter mechanisms.

Detrusor instability

This accounts for about two-thirds of cases and is also called 'unstable bladder' incontinence. In this condition the uninhibited detrusor contractions result in the bladder neck mechanism failing, leading to the distal urethral mechanism also failing and incontinence resulting.

The incontinence episodes may be reported by the relatives as 'willful' — typically the person had been on the toilet for ten minutes, went into the living room and then incontinence occurred. After diagnosis the cause (involuntary contractions triggered by many things — movement, coughing, volume of urine, etc.) must be carefully explained. The diagnosis, however, is best made after urodynamic studies, though the confused and/or severely immobile patient should not be subjected to these investigations without appropriate consultation.

Overflow incontinence

The commonest cause in both sexes is a loaded

rectum. In men, prostate enlargement is also a common factor. A constant dribble of urine is a frequently described symptom and it is then mandatory to examine the abdomen for a distended bladder and do a rectal examination. Women go into retention less easily than men. In addition to constipation, a pelvic mass should be excluded. Drugs (anticholinergics) can cause retention, as can urethral strictures (often post-catheter or surgical trauma).

Prostatism

This common condition of elderly men presents with a history of delay in the start of micturition and a poor stream with terminal dribbling. Sufferers may be incontinent due to *urgency* (75 per cent of patients also have some evidence of detrusor instability), *overflow* (if they have gone into retention) and *post-micturition dribble* (PMD). This is an exaggerated form of a condition that affects most men of all ages (the leakage of small amounts of urine after micturition has ceased). When prostatism is not a problem PMD can be avoided. At the end of micturition the scrotal sac should be lifted gently and the base of the urethra gently pushed upon, to allow a few extra millilitres of urine to be passed.

Neurogenic bladder

Damage to the innervation of the bladder and cortical damage can lead to a neurogenic bladder (see Table 22.3). There is usually a lack of awareness and voiding occurs automatically once a certain volume has been reached. Some patients, however, learn to control voiding by increasing their intra-abdominal pressure.

Table 22.3 Causes of neurogenic bladder

Uninhibited neurogenic bladder
Cerebrovascular disease (multi infarct dementia or stroke)
Frontal lobe tumour (precipitant micturition)
Parkinson's disease
Normal pressure hydrocephalus

Reflex neurogenic bladder
Spinal cord disease (disc prolapse, spinal cord tumour, etc.)

Atonic neurogenic bladder
Diabetes mellitus
Tabes dorsalis

Investigations

Not every patient requires a full work-up, including invasive bladder studies. Usually the diagnosis is clear once a basic history and examination, coupled with a continence chart, have been completed (see Table 22.4). If the problem appears complex (e.g. there are elements of stress and urge incontinence), then referral to a urodynamic clinic is often worthwhile.

Table 22.4 Investigative process

History
Medication (diuretics, laxatives, tranquillizers)
Medical and surgical history

Examination
Mental state, mobility, neurological examination, PR,PV,abdominal examination

Investigations
Continence chart,MSU, blood sugar, U&E; and possibly: plain abdominal x-ray, U/S, KUB (kidney, ureter, bladder), IVU, TPHA/VDRL, cystometry — urodynamics

Treatment

Antibiotics should be used to treat a urinary tract infection (>1000 WBC and >1.0 million colony count). If associated with a catheter this should be removed, albeit temporarily. If there are accompanying systemic symptoms and signs (e.g. confusion, hypotension and rigors) then parenteral antibiotics should be used. Precipitating causes of urinary incontinence, such as drugs, should be altered where possible. Outflow tract obstruction can be managed conservatively in some selected cases (severe frailty, personal choice) by the use of a long-term catheter. Most other cases benefit from referral to a specialist Urologist. Gynaecological advice should be sought in patients with a uterine prolapse, cystocoele and atrophic vaginitis (the latter is usually helped markedly by the application of oestrogen cream).

The ward environment (clearly marked toilets) and mobility exercises assist patients greatly. Confused patients may be helped by reality orientation techniques. Praise and the short-term use of a two-hourly toileting regimen should begin the process of assessment. Hourly toileting is difficult and the charts fail to be filled in after a few days. The chart should provide a 'pattern' and help with diagnosis and management, and not become an end in itself.

A few people with unstable bladders may derive limited benefit from anticholinergic drugs (e.g. flavoxate). Emepronium bromide (Cetiprin), a quaternary ammonium compound, causes mucosal ulceration in the oesophagus and elsewhere, is very poorly absorbed, and should not be used. The use of anticholinergics is not without risk of side-effects, and as their benefits are usually minimal, careful consideration should be given to their use (especially their continued use) if improvement does not occur.

Catheters have their uses, intermittently for some, permanently for a carefully selected group of patients where there is also user acceptance and satisfaction. Acutely ill people often need catheterizing, though it should be removed at the earliest opportunity in the rehabilitation process. Catheters should never be used for ease of nursing/caring but only if the patient also benefits. There is a vast range of different catheter types, and all advice on continence aids, their use, selection, comfort and suitability should be sought from a continence adviser.

Pads have reduced the laundry problems of people with persistent incontinence and are now widely used. Most, however, are only able to cope with a dribble of urine rather than an intense void of half a litre. Better, more absorbent pads cost more, and most health authorities are finding that bills for pads are escalating, so the range of pads available may be limited. It is usual for most people with persistent incontinence to use pads in preference to regular trips to the toilet. Pads tend to give a feeling of security, particularly on long journeys. Pads have certainly reduced the use of indwelling catheters in institutions and have probably reduced the risks of septicaemia and death due to catheter-related infections.

FAECAL INCONTINENCE

Faecal incontinence is far less common than urinary incontinence but much less well tolerated and by its nature a cause of great distress to both patient and carer. There are three main groups of causes (Table 22.5).

Table 22.5 Causes of faecal incontinence

Bowel disease
Carcinoma of colon/rectum
Diverticular disease
Ischaemic bowel
Ulcerative colitis/proctocolitis
Diabetic neuropathy
Laxative abuse

Faecal overloading/impaction

Neurogenic bowel
Dementing syndromes
Normal pressure hydrocephalus
Spinal cord disease

The overwhelming number of cases are due to faecal overloading/impaction, resulting either in solid stool being passed involuntarily, or in *diarrhoea* (spurious) due to the impaction extending back up the colon and liquid stool seeping past. Disimpaction may initially need manual removal, followed by enemas. Stimulants (e.g. senna) should never be given until the lower bowel and rectum has been cleared as their use can cause colic and precipitate subacute and acute obstruction.

Investigation and management

In all cases a rectal examination must be carried out and a sigmoidoscopy considered. If the rectum is empty a plain abdominal x-ray will confirm a diagnosis of high faecal overloading. A rectal examination will confirm impaction and help exclude a rectal carcinoma which can impair rectal tone. Also, conditions which inhibit defaecation through fear of pain during a bowel movement (e.g. haemorrhoids or fissure) will be revealed.

Diarrhoea may need investigating further, by including stool specimens and rectal biopsy. Other bowel disease may need investigating via barium enema or colonoscopy. Diarrhoea (from whatever cause) can cause incontinence in any age group. Neurogenic bowel (with similar aetiologies to the bladder condition) is usually diagnosed from the history. Manometry studies are available in some research centres. People suffering from dementia syndromes may have voluntary incontinence if they cannot find the toilet. At the end stage of the disease they may lose higher control of the bowels and bladder. Constipating drugs (codeine phosphate) accompanied by regular enemas can stop the involuntary passage of faeces.

Excessive consumption of laxatives can cause faecal incontinence. This abuse may be suspected by the biochemical findings of hypokalaemia, melanosis coli (black mucosal discoloration) on sigmoidoscopy and the fact that the laxatives are kept hidden.

An active and energetic approach will enable many patients to regain continence. For the person who does not, a sympathetic and enlightened approach is essential. In a well-managed environment overt evidence of urinary or faecal incontinence should be unacceptable.

Key points

- Incontinence is an involuntary loss of urine or faeces in an inappropriate place.

- To be continent an elderly person must be mobile, be able to find the toilet, be appropriately clothed for the journey and use a suitably designed toilet.
- History and examination includes rectal, vaginal and urine microscopy and culture.
- Causes of incontinence of urine include infection, stress incontinence, detrusor instability, overflow, prostatism, neurogenic bladder, uterine prolapse, cystocoele and atrophic vaginitis.
- Limited benefit is derived from drug usage in urinary incontinence.
- Urinary catheters may be used intermittently or permanently.
- Causes of faecal incontinence include bowel disease (carcinoma of rectum, diverticular disease, laxative abuse), faecal overloading and impaction and neurogenic bowel.
- The overwhelming number of cases of faecal incontinence are due to faecal overloading/ impaction.
- Stimulant laxatives should never be given until the lower bowel has been cleared. Investigation and management of faecal incontinence includes history, examination, PR, sigmoidoscopy and laxative review.

FURTHER READING

Brocklehurst JC. Treatment of constipation and faecal incontinence in old people. *Practitioner* 1964; **193**:779–782.

Brocklehurst JC (ed.). *Urology in the Elderly.* Churchill Livingstone, Edinburgh, 1984.

Castleden CM, Duffin HM. (1981) Guidelines for controlling urinary incontinence without drugs or catheters. *Age Ageing* 1981; **10**:186–190.

Mandelstrom D. *Incontinence.* Disabled Living Foundation, London, 1977.

Percy JP, Neill ME, Kandiah TK, Swash M. A neurogenic factor in faecal incontinence in the elderly. *Age Ageing* 1982; **11**:175–179.

23 PRESSURE SORES

- Prevalence
- History and aetiology
- Blood flow and oxygen
- Pathology
- Healing
- Prevention
- Treating existing sores

Necrosis of skin, adipose tissue and muscle caused by pressure occurs rapidly in acutely and chronically ill elderly people. Necrosis of any other tissue (e.g. myocardial infarction) leads to considerable medical attention, whereas death of skin and muscle overlying hips and buttocks — often caused by and causing whole body complications — attracts very little notice. This state of affairs is changing for many reasons; increasing awareness of medical responsibility, medical audit, scientific research, cost management and the new spectre of litigation being a few. Some groups of people appear especially at risk (see Table 23.1).

Table 23.1 Groups at risk of pressure sores

Acutely and chronically ill elderly
Neurological disease (stroke, Alzheimer's disease, Parkinson's disease, multiple sclerosis)
Spinal cord injury
During and after orthopaedic surgery
Postoperatively (general surgery)
The very ill (ITU all ages)
The dying.

PREVALENCE

Large-scale studies in the 1970s indicated a prevalence rate of about 9 per cent of all UK hospital patients with some form of pressure sore. This contrasted with about 5 per cent in Scandinavian research. However, more recent data indicate that the UK range is wide (2.7 to 66.0 per cent), the highest figures occurring in the elderly with fractured femurs. The lowest figures come from units where dedicated individuals apply education and resources to considerable patient benefit. The total cost to the health service in purely financial terms is enormous, each health district spending close to 1 million pounds per year on treating this one condition.

HISTORY AND AETIOLOGY

Pressure sores are not a new phenomenon. The earliest reference concerns an Egyptian twelfthdynasty Priestess of Amen. When unwrapped following her arrival at the British Museum she was noted to have a sacral pressure sore (which had presumably occurred whilst she was ill and dying thousands of years ago). Her claim to immortal fame continues in that her pressure sore was covered with a piece of gazelle skin, making her the first known recipient of a skin graft. There are Biblical references to pressure sores (Isaiah) and subsequently all the great names in medicine (Quesnay, Fabriscius, Brown-Sequard, Charcot) wrote learnedly on the subject. Many of their themes carry through to current thoughts on aetiology (see Table 23.2).

Table 23.2 Causes of pressure sores

Intrinsic causes
Paralysis
Decreased sensation (reduced pain stimuli)
Decreased attention (sedation, coma, depression)
Diminished tissue turgor (dehydration, hypotension)
Malnutrition
Peripheral vascular disease
Systemic disease
Failure of vasomotor reflexes (recent cord injury)
Endothelial cell disruption in ill patients (compared with
   healthy patients).

Extrinsic causes
The application of pressure:
   Long periods on hard trolleys
   Relative hardness of hospital beds
   Long periods up in a chair
Macerated skin secondary to sweat and incontinence
Shearing forces — in bed and during poor lifting/turning

BLOOD FLOW AND OXYGEN

The mean capillary pressure (in healthy medical students) is approximately 25 mmHg. We have no measurements for elderly people let alone those who are ill. Beyond 25 mmHg the blood vessels are occluded and the surrounding tissues (including skin) become anoxic. Pressure loading studies show that healthy people can tolerate high pressures for short periods very well, their oxygen-carrying capacity in the tissues recovering from the 'assault'. The studies conclude that the amount of damage is proportional to the product of the pressure and the time for which it is applied, but in the at-risk groups the amount of pressure and duration of time before damage occurs is probably very short. A bed-ridden patient easily generates pressures in excess of 100 mmHg

especially over the sacrum, heels and greater trochanters (96 per cent of pressure sores occur below the umbilicus).

PATHOLOGY

Eighty per cent of sores are superficial (type 1) and 20 per cent are deep (type 2).

Figure 23.1 Superficial (type 1) pressure sore

Superficial (Fig. 23.1). These sores occur mainly in dehydrated and incontinent patients exposed to sustained pressure (most commonly seen postoperatively). The majority of these sores are preventable. They will deepen if pressure is not relieved. Histologically the endothelial cell lining is swollen but remains intact.

Deep (Fig. 23.2). These are formed when localized high pressure cuts off a wedge-shaped area of tissue usually adjacent to a bony prominence (see Fig 23.3).

Microthrombi block the capillaries and the endothelial cell lining separates, allowing extensive inflammatory damage to occur. The necrotic tissue breaks down over days to form a deep sore.

HEALING

Once pressure is relieved and the blood supply to surrounding tissues restored, most sores heal by the following processes.

Debridement. Over a few weeks the necrotic slough (often hardened to form a scab/eschar) separates from the wound. This occurs naturally and should rarely be interfered with.

Contraction. Over the next month the wound contracts and this forms one of the most important

Figure 23.2 Deep (type 2) pressure sore

aspects of the closure of the pressure sore. To contract fully the wound needs to be moist and free from infection.

Epithelialization. Epithelial cells migrate from the ulcer margin (healthy skin), but this is decreased by dryness, infection, systemic disease and by some topical agents.

Remodelling. There is early profuse growth of capillaries which diminishes as scar collagen matures and subsequent fibrosis leaves a depressed scar.

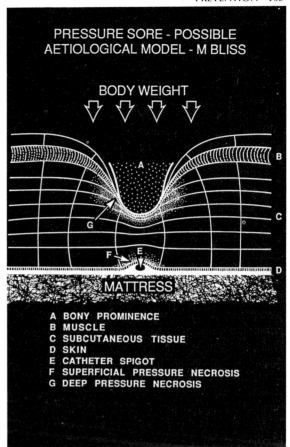

Figure 23.3 Possible aetiological model of a pressure sore (M. Bliss)

PREVENTION

All patients in the at-risk groups should have anti-pressure protection starting immediately a new illness or injury (at home or in hospital) occurs. Nurses use assessment scales (Norton, Waterlow and Braden) to try to predict potential risk. At home, pillows can be used to protect bony prominences and the patient should be repositioned frequently. Alternating-pressure air mattresses (APAMs) such as the *large-cell ripple mattress* can be used for short-term protection.

Hospital admission (from A&E to discharge planning) requires at-risk patients to have their pressure areas actively managed. The most effective medium-priced APAM available in the UK is the **Pegasus Airwave mattress** (see Fig. 23.4), a semi-portable system. The Pegasus mattress has a double bank of air cells that provide alternating pressure relief so that no area is subject to ischaemia for more than a few minutes. In most cases this mattress obviates the need for regular turning.

Static air mattresses, flotation beds and other low-pressure mattresses and beds all have considerable disadvantages. Patients should have bed cradles in place and may benefit from an anchored fleece at the end of the bed. Immobile patients should have a

Figure 23.4 The Pegasus Airwave mattress

pillow between the knees. Ill patients should be nursed in bed and then, as they recover, sit out for gradually increasing periods.

TREATING EXISTING SORES

Local treatment

Local hyperaemia is common, as is a raised white cell count with associated mild pyrexia. Debridement should occur naturally, aided by cleaning the wound with saline and keeping it moist (with one of the numerous non-toxic dressings). Antiseptics such as Eusol should be avoided. Deep wounds should not be packed but the opinion of a plastic surgeon sought early. Heel blisters are best left exposed until dry and less inflamed.

General measures

Other medical conditions (e.g. diabetes, dehydration) need to be treated vigorously, and in the initial stages pain relief is usually necessary, some patients needing regular low-dose morphine. Patients may need catheterizing for a short while to ensure that the sore is kept clean and dry. Offensive odours should be tackled with increased frequency of dressings, charcoal-containing coverings and occasionally metronidazole (via suppository). This should help stop the patient becoming depressed and from being ostracised by other patients and staff.

A normal diet with supplements if necessary is usually sufficient, though some patients may require supplementary feeding and advice from the dietitian and/or nutrition team. Subclinical scurvy is quite common in the elderly and vitamin C is necessary for wound healing (1 g a day in the healing phase). Other vitamin deficiencies should be sought and treated. Patients with chronic sores often develop an anaemia that is unresponsive to haematinics, and the patient and the rate of ulcer healing benefit from a packed-cell blood transfusion. Drug therapy should be reviewed to try to stop or decrease corticosteroids and other anti-inflammatory drugs (NSAIDs, etc.) which delay wound healing. There is some evidence that zinc-deficient people have poor wound healing, and as zinc is difficult to measure it can be given empirically (as zinc sulphate 220 mg bd) in the healing phase.

As the patient improves and begins to mobilize, most sores heal rapidly. Mobility increases muscle bulk and blood flow, decreases oedema and all these measures enhance ulcer healing.

Surgery

A surgical opinion should be sought in all cases where a deep sore is present and not healing rapidly. Modern anaesthetic and plastic surgery techniques (myoplasty) have revolutionized the care in this type of case. Rapid surgery has the added advantage of allowing the elderly person to leave hospital quickly, avoiding months of slow medical treatment and possible further complications.

Key points

- At-risk groups include the frail elderly, those with spinal cord injury or neurological disease, and patients who are very ill or dying.
- Prevalence rates vary but approximately 8 per cent is a consistent norm.

- Health districts spend about £1 million per year treating pressure sores.
- Aetiology includes both intrinsic and extrinsic causes.
- Damage = pressure × time.
- Pressure sores are either superficial (80 per cent) or deep (20 per cent).
- Healing comprises debridement, contraction, epithelialization and remodelling.
- Most superficial sores would be prevented if all ill elderly people were nursed on APAMs (alternating-pressure air mattresses) and had bed cradles in place.
- General treatment measures include pain relief, nutrition assessment, the management of other medical problems and attention to continence and mobility.
- Pressure sores are as much a medical as nursing responsibility.

FURTHER READING

Bader D (ed.). *Pressure Sores: Clinical Practice and Scientific Approach.* Macmillan, New York, 1990.

Barton AA, Barton N. *The Management and Prevention of Pressure Sores.* Faber, London, 1981.

Kenedi RM, Cowden JM, Scales JT (eds). *Bedsore Biomechanics.* Macmillan, London, 1976.

Kosiak M. Etiology and pathology of ischaemic ulcers. *Arch Phys Med Rehabil* 1959; **40**:62–69.

24 ACCIDENTAL HYPOTHERMIA

- Definition
- Occurrence
- Regulation of body temperature
- Clinical features
- Management
- Preventive measures

DEFINITION

Accidental hypothermia is defined as a core body temperature below 35°C. The core or central temperature is reflected accurately when measured *with a low reading thermometer* in the oesophagus, the covered external auditory meatus, or (more commonly) the rectum. Oral temperature readings are unreliable. The temperature of *immediately* voided urine can be used to reflect the central/core temperature. The hypothermia is termed 'accidental' to differentiate it from the carefully induced hypothermia of some surgical procedures. It is a medical emergency with a high morbidity and mortality.

OCCURRENCE

In the early 1960s reports began appearing in the medical press of isolated cases of accidental hypothermia. Researchers, including the Royal College of Physicians, studied this and found a true phenomenon occurring. One large study involving the elderly at home found few cases of actual hypothermia but almost 10 per cent with very low core temperatures just outside the definition range. This prehypothermic group appeared to have some social characteristics in common — including poverty. Extrapolation from this study indicated that nearly 750 000 elderly people were at risk of hypothermia, but large long-term follow-up studies have not been done to confirm the size of the problem or the extent of the risk.

The occurrence of accidental hypothermia is usually related to a low environmental temperature — hence it is especially common in winter. It is not unusual to hear stories of elderly people getting out of bed, falling, and remaining on the floor for several hours. They are usually poorly clothed with no heating in the room and are only discovered 24–48 hours later by friends, neighbours or statutory services. However, cases can occur when a person is in bed and, although apparently well covered, not generating sufficient body heat, the insulation obviously being ineffective. Accidental hypothermia cases can therefore also be found in hospitals and residential homes.

REGULATION OF BODY TEMPERATURE

The maintenance of a constant central temperature of 37°C is under nervous system control with afferent and efferent pathways. On exposure to cold, heat is conserved by cutaneous vasoconstriction and increased heat produced by shivering. Appreciation of cold at a conscious level encourages movement away from the cold environment, the wearing of suitable clothing and occasionally exercise. Most elderly people have normal thermoregulatory mechanisms, but there is an at-risk subgroup where some degree of thermoregulatory failure occurs and where the mechanisms for conserving body heat are impaired. These subjects, while their deep body temperature is falling, have a poor shivering response, are less aware of the cold exposure, and tend not to complain of the cold or alter their environment.

Drugs

Drugs such as alcohol, sedatives and tranquillizers can act on the nervous system and further impair the physiological mechanisms. Phenothiazines (e.g. chlorpromazine) affect temperature regulation by abolishing the shivering response and causing vasodilatation. They also lessen the awareness to environmental changes and hazards. Alcohol, sedatives, tranquillizers, hypnotics and antidepressants have all been implicated in causing cases of accidental hypothermia. Nitrazepam (a benzodiazepine with an extremely long half-life) can have accumulation problems causing drowsiness, ataxia and falls which in some circumstances can predispose to a hypothermic state.

Clinical disorders

The most severe cases of hypothermia usually have some underlying clinical condition (see Table 24.1).

CLINICAL FEATURES

All organ systems of the body are affected and with increasing severity as the core temperature falls

Table 24.1 Clinical conditions associated with hypothermia

Endocrine	Hypothyroidism Hypopituitarism
Vascular	Stroke Transient ischaemic attack
Neurological	Epilepsy
Immobility	Severe arthritis Parkinson's disease Paraplegia/hemiplegia Fractures
Psychiatric	Depression Drug overdosage Chronic confusional states e.g. dementia syndromes
Severe infections/ circulatory disturbances	Bronchopneumonia Myocardial infarction Pulmonary embolism
Unconscious patient	Postoperative Sedated Diabetic

Table 24.2 Clinical features of hypothermia

Skin	Cold, marble-like, pallor, subcutaneous oedema (causing puffiness)
Neurological	Confusion, disorientation, drowsiness and coma. Ataxia, flapping tremor, extensor plantars. Reflexes slow and then become absent (incl. pupillary)
Muscular	Stiffen then hypertonic (can simulate meningism)
CVS	Poor volume pulse, slowing to atrial fibrillation or sinus bradycardia
Respiratory	Respirations become slower and shallower
GI	Paralytic ileus, gastric dilatation and acute pancreatitis can occur. Insulin is inactivated
Renal	Decrease in renal plasma flow, GFR. Oliguria occurs
Haematological	Venous blood pools and is unreliable for sampling. There is a decrease in arterial oxygen saturation

(see Table 24.2). The skin feels cold and may become mottled and feel like marble. If clinical examination reveals a cool/cold abdomen or inner thigh then always suspect hypothermia. Intense peripheral vasoconstriction gives extreme pallor to the skin and the face becomes puffy as a result of subcutaneous oedema. This and a husky voice (if the patient is conscious) due to oedema and poor movement of the vocal cords often lead to a mistaken diagnosis of hypothyroidism. A body orifice such as the rectum or mouth may feel cold and shivering is absent.

Figure 24.1 The top trace shows the normal PQRST complex; the bottom trace shows the 'J' wave at the junction of the QRS and ST segments

As the core temperature falls so cerebration slows. Below 32°C there is usually confusion and disorientation, eventually leading to drowsiness and coma. As body fat cools the abdomen takes on a 'doughy' feel. Muscles stiffen and become hypertonic (giving rise to neck stiffness simulating meningism). Ataxia is common, an involuntary flapping tremor may be seen and plantar responses become extensor. Reflexes are slowed and then absent (including the pupillary response), the knee jerks characteristically being the last reflexes to disappear. Respirations become slow and shallow and there is a fall in arterial oxygen saturation. The pulse is of poor volume and may be difficult to find. The rhythm changes to slow atrial fibrillation or sinus bradycardia owing to the effect of the cold on the atrial pacemaker. The heart sounds eventually become inaudible. The blood pressure falls and is then difficult to measure. A pathognomonic ECG feature is the 'J' wave best seen in lead 1 (see Fig. 24.1).

Cardiac failure can occur, as can gastric dilatation with the risk of aspiration. Acute pancreatitis is relatively common (the pancreas being very sensitive to the effects of the cold) though the diagnosis is difficult. Paralytic ileus occurs, and a decrease in renal plasma flow and glomerular filtration rate with oliguria is common. Venous blood tends to pool and hence for accuracy arterial samples must be taken. Tissue metabolism and oxygen consumption are decreased. Insulin is inactivated by very low temperatures and hence glucose cannot enter cells. Abnormal glucose measurements are common; however, on rewarming glucose rapidly enters tissues and hypoglycaemia can result.

MANAGEMENT

Mild degrees of hypothermia (around 35°C) can occasionally be treated at home, but associated medical problems and adverse social circumstances usually preclude this. All other degrees of hypothermia require urgent hospital admission. Some doctors believe that practically all hypothermia patients should be managed in intensive care, others that most intervention is unwarranted and even dangerous. Intensive nursing can be, and for the majority is, performed on ordinary wards. The management must take into account the metabolic, cardiac and biochemical problems that can occur. An airway may

Table 24.3 Categories during rewarming (after Maclean and Emslie Smith)

Favourable
Rewarming spontaneously and rapidly 0.5°C/hour
No haemodynamic complications
Consciousness steadily recovers
Biochemical and haematological abnormalities correct
    themselves

Less favourable
Unexpected hypotension ('rewarming collapse')
Episodic sinus bradycardia or AV block
Profound hypoglycaemia
Persistent hypoxaemia
Intercurrent infection

Poor prognosis
Severe bronchopneumonia
Circulatory/cardiac arrest
Acute pancreatitis

Worst prognosis
Core temperature fails to rise, or rises only very slowly
Evidence of 'shock'

need to be established, fluid and electrolytes or acid–base balance may need to be corrected, and the heart and vital signs monitored. Most patients fall into one of four categories during rewarming (see Table 24.3).

The 'less favourable' category probably accounts for the largest number of patients seen clinically. A few points should be made concerning cardiac arrest. At low temperatures the decreased oxygen demands permit longer periods of arrest with theoretical eventual recovery; however, electrical defibrillation is usually unsuccessful at temperatures below 30°C and some patients have underlying disease of such severity that cardiac resuscitation is inappropriate.

Figure 24.2 Space blanket

ANTICIPATING AND AVOIDING COMPLICATIONS

A plain chest x-ray may detect pneumonia or pulmonary oedema (there can be marked fluid shifts from one compartment to another). Similarly, abdominal x-rays may show bowel dilatation or free gas, indicating ileus or perforation. Blood sampling (*arterial*) may suggest infection, kidney disease, glucose intolerance, pancreatitis, or hypothyroidism. Blood gases (corrected for temperature) may be necessary. ECG or cardiac monitoring may show dysrhythmias, etc.

Many of the complications (fluid shifts, hypoxia, hypercalcaemia and metabolic acidosis) may correct themselves during the rewarming process. The rate and means of rewarming is controversial (slow peripheral, fast peripheral, or central rewarming). The ambient temperature for those admitted should be between 25 and 30°C. At this temperature (most easily achieved in a side room with heaters) most patients rewarm spontaneously at about 0.5–1.0°C/hour if insulated against further heat loss (using a 'space blanket'; see Fig 24.2). The patient should be placed into the blanket (silver-side-up if only silvered on one side) and swaddled; that is, the head should be included to prevent the massive heat loss from this

area. The rectal temperature should be monitored, ideally continuously with an electrical temperature probe.

Maclean and Emslie-Smith have formulated the idea of a conservative management plan. A modified version is shown in Table 24.4.

Table 24.4 A management plan for hypothermia

1. Nurse in ambient temperature 25–32°C
2. Ripple mattress/space blanket
3. Cardiac monitor, portable chest x-ray
4. IV loading-dose prophylactic antibiotics (after urine, sputum and blood cultures)
5. Monitor rectal temperature, respiration rate and blood pressure
6. Monitor arterial blood gases (give oxygen if necessary)
7. Monitor blood glucose, electrolytes, acid–base balance
8. IV access but no routine infusions, steroids, vasoactive drugs or thyroid hormone
9. Disturb as little as possible

For most patients slow external rewarming is the best method despite the fact that it means prolonging the physiological abnormality for many hours. Hospital staff are conversant with it, and — importantly — survival figures equate with those of the more complicated rapid rewarming techniques. 'Rewarming collapse' is severe hypotension, probably as a result of rewarming too fast causing a sudden fall in peripheral resistance. Cooling the patient again usually stabilizes the blood pressure and a slower rewarming regimen then employed. Occasionally inotropes can be given to 'support' the blood pressure while more active rewarming occurs. Rapid central rewarming techniques (gastric/colonic lavage, warm IV infusions, mediastinal irrigation) have been used in specialist centres.

PREVENTIVE MEASURES

Many elderly people can be considered at risk from hypothermia. A pattern recognition should emerge among GPs, health visitors, district nurses and non-statutory workers, involving the *social factors* (poor financial resources, poor heating, inadequate accommodation, inadequate clothing, outside lavatory, poor lighting, dependent on statutory services, recent bereavement etc.) and the *medical factors* (undernutrition, chronic confusion, sedative medication, associated diseases, etc.) that indicate high risk.

General practitioners and district nurses must have adequate access to low-reading thermometers to diagnose cases early and if possible avoid hospital admission. Many local authorities and non-statutory groups such as Age Concern or Help the Aged run winter hypothermia schemes, giving better access to warmer clothing, extra heaters, and advice. Good-neighbour schemes in very bad weather can help enormously by the provision of a hot meal or drink and a close eye kept on the situation.

Governmental responses have been inadequate. Many elderly people cite poverty for not spending extra money on heating, clothing and food. The elderly should not be reliant on pitifully low (and complicated to assess) 'severe weather payments', or indeed have to take out loans from Social Services. An adequate pension would be all that most require.

General advice from any source on food, clothing, bedding and household features needs to be more widespread and comprehensive. For maximum comfort and warmth, clothing needs to be light, loose and loosely woven with a few layers to trap air. The same applies to bed-clothing (though duvets are extremely warm and useful). A hat and warm socks should be worn in bed. Electric overblankets are excellent, but the use of heated underblankets is not advised if there is any problem with incontinence. If the bed abuts on an outside wall it should be moved. In severe weather consideration should be given to one-room living, even to the provision of a commode in that room if the passage to and from the toilet is unheated.

There should be a store of carbohydrate-rich foods to be used in the event of an emergency, and some spare blankets on the floor in case a fall occurs. Techniques can be taught for getting up off the floor after a fall.

The true mortality statistics for hypothermia are difficult to assess because of low reporting (if written on a death certificate it implies neglect and hence a Coroner's inquest is necessary). Many casualties are not found until many days after the event, making an accurate diagnosis impossible. Most cases could be prevented and a pre-winter assessment of medical and social factors could help considerably.

Key points

- Accidental hypothermia is defined as a core body temperature below 35°C.
- Core or central body temperature must be measured with a low-reading thermometer (oesophagus, external auditory meatus, rectum).
- The occurrence of accidental hypothermia is usually related to a low environmental temperature.
- Most elderly people have normal thermoregulatory mechanisms.
- Drugs can impair the physiological responses to cold and predispose to hypothermia.
- The most severe cases of hypothermia usually have some underlying clinical condition.
- All organ systems of the body are affected with some unique clinical features.
- Management of established cases requires rewarming in hospital.
- Rewarming complications (e.g. hypotension) are common.
- Preventive measures include assessing for the social and medical predisposing causes.
- General advice includes information on nutrition, clothing (many loose layers, wear hat and socks in bed), bedding, house heating and emergency measures.

FURTHER READING

Maclean D, Emslie-Smith D. *Accidental Hypothermia.* Blackwell Scientific, Oxford, 1977.

Maudgal D. *Hypothermia: Medical and Social Aspects.* Pergamon Press, Oxford, 1987.

Wicks M. *Old and Cold: Hypothermia and Social Policy.* Heinemann, London, 1978.

25 JOINT CONTRACTURES

- Immobility
- Common causes of immobility leading to contractures
- Prevention and management

This dreadful condition, though seen less frequently, is still too common in units dealing with the chronically disabled. When putting the elderly to bed for long periods was a common treatment the sight of numerous skeletal figures in the fetal position with hips, knees and elbows contracted, stress fractures and pressure sores on opposing limbs must have saddened everyone. It is hard to believe, but nonetheless true, that this state arose from putting the sick elderly to bed for too long. One of the slogans of the first generation of geriatricians was 'bed is bad'. This message has been taken up but often with too much zeal and too little thought. Being up in a chair when ill may be totally inappropriate, as long periods spent immobile in a chair results in a chair-shaped person. This is only marginally less of an evil.

IMMOBILITY

Synovial joints must move to remain healthy, for immobility produces damaging effects in the joint and the surrounding tissues. Bone, cartilage, muscle, ligaments and synovium are all affected. It appears that the water and proteoglycan gel cushioning the collagen fibres is reduced, leading to friction between the fibres and the development of adhesions. Increased and abnormal collagen cross-linking at the molecular level also occurs, changing its tensile properties.

The effects of immobility on joints have been studied using animal models. A proliferation of fibro-fatty connective tissue covers the entire inner surface of the joint within 30 days of immobility. During the second month the connective tissue becomes more dense and adherent with the surface cartilage becoming thin and irregular. The degree of cartilage damage depends on the rigidity of immobilization, the position and any compressive force. Compression results in erosion of cartilage and bone. If the immobilization is continued, the underlying marrow becomes hyperaemic as vascular connective tissue proliferates, penetrating the subchondral bone producing bone cysts. Similar changes are seen in neglected long-standing contractures in patients. The bones forming the joints may be shown on x-ray to have fused together.

COMMON CAUSES OF IMMOBILITY LEADING TO CONTRACTURES

Joint pain

Inflammation (secondary to infection, rheumatoid disease, injury, osteoarthritis, gout, etc.) leads to pain and muscle spasm, producing immobility. If prolonged this produces disuse muscle and bone atrophy, further compounding the immobility.

Spasticity

Following a cerebrovascular accident or in other neurological conditions (e.g. multiple sclerosis), hypertonic muscles of large bulk overcome their antagonists to produce a joint held in an abnormal posture. Prolonged spasticity is associated with derangement of muscle spindles and inappropriate inhibition of the antagonist muscles which may make the deformity worse. Eventually this situation leads to fixed shortening of the muscles involved.

Fetal posture

Patients with advanced dementia syndromes (and some people deprived of sensory input) may adopt a curled-up position in bed, obviously resenting all interference. Attempts to improve posture are usually resisted (with unexpected vigour) and fail.

Burns

The contractures resulting from burns involve a different aetiological mechanism. They are a result of wound healing and subsequent contraction involving contractile myofibroblasts (cells not present in the other causes). However, inadequate changing of position may result in oedema and pressure ulceration of the skin with subsequent infection. Management consists of firm pressure around healing/grafted burns to control oedema and prevent contractures.

PREVENTION AND MANAGEMENT

In 1843, W.J. Little gave a lecture and clinical demonstration entitled 'Deformities of the Human Frame'. He noted that spastic contractures are more difficult to treat than others, particularly in the upper limbs. He used springs and splints to aid deficient muscles, and he instructed his nurses to endeavour to straighten the affected joints several times a day. Over 150 years later it is still possible for elderly patients to receive less attention than this.

Joint pain

The inflammatory process must be attacked with all the methods at our disposal. These include aspiration to confirm the diagnosis and to relieve a tense 'hot' joint; drugs; and physical methods — for example, heat and ice and, paradoxically, the temporary immobilization of joints in good functional postures by

Figure 25.1 'Cricket-pad' type of orthotic splint

means of orthotics (splints), particularly at night. Active or assisted exercises are used to regain muscle power, encourage reabsorption of effusions and regain range of movement. Early contractures (when an elderly person has been confined to bed with an

Figure 25.2 Correct positioning of a stroke patient (see text)

intercurrent illness) respond to energetic treatment with analgesics, active exercises and passive stretching (manually or with traction). Injection of local anaesthetic can help reduce pain and spasm and allow treatment programmes to begin. Rarely manipulation under sedation or anaesthesia is required (there is a real risk of fracturing bones during manipulation under anaesthesia and it requires expert assessment). Any gain in range of movement should be maintained and in some cases splints are used. Splints can be made of Plaster of Paris, but increasingly light thermoplastic materials are being used. Velcro fastenings aid easy removal for active exercises, but strongly resisting joints may need serial splinting using the 'cricket-pad' type of orthotic with firmer side-straps and buckles (see Fig. 25.1). Progress is often slow and can cause discomfort. Pressure sore formation must be assiduously avoided. However, serial splinting can

result in improved function and the regained use of an otherwise painful, contracted and useless limb.

Spasticity

The prevention of spastic contractures depends on good positioning of the patient combined with frequent gentle exercising of the limbs through a normal range of movements. Physiotherapists are the 'experts' in this field and nurses and doctors should take guidance from them. In the case of a stroke patient the limbs should be placed in the opposite position to the fully developed spastic posture (see Fig. 25.2). Thus elbows and wrists are extended, fingers are abducted and extended. A bed cradle should keep the bed-clothes from actively extending the feet. During the initial flaccid stage of a stroke, care must be taken not to stretch joint capsules (particularly the shoulder) by traction on the joint during lifting and positioning of the patient. The positioning diagram should be by the patient's bed so that the less experienced can refer to it. The shoulder or 'Australian lift' method is used to move the patient (see Fig. 25.3).

After a few days spasticity begins to develop (the time scale is variable and in some cases the limbs remain flaccid). All joints need to be put through a normal range of movements several times a day; this can be whenever the patient is turned, cleaned or examined. Sudden or jerky movements can induce clonus (rhythmic beating movements) and should be avoided. Slow sustained traction will reduce tone for several minutes, and by using postural reflexes involv-

Figure 25.3 The 'Australian' lift carried out by two helpers

ing the neck and trunk tone in the limbs may be reduced to allow an improved range of movement. Ice, vibration or tapping may be used by the therapists to reduce tone during treatment. As soon as power begins to return, active movements, assisted if necessary by slings and counterweights, are used. Exercises involving symmetrical movements of the limbs (e.g. the Bobath technique) which can be practised by the patient at any time are particularly valuable. The full range of therapy expertise, including hydrotherapy if possible, should be brought to bear to prevent poor posture and contractures. Drug therapy can play a role. Drugs specifically aimed at reducing excess spasticity are available (e.g. Baclofen/lioresal and Dantrolene/sodium dantrium), but confusional states in the frail elderly can be a side-effect. Analgesia plus low-dose oral diazepam (used as a muscle relaxant) is another useful combination.

Spastic contractures which have been present for months are very difficult to treat. Surgical treatment is only usually appropriate for a small number of patients with specific problems. For example, lengthening of the Achilles tendon may be necessary to overcome severe equinus deformity (if stretching under anaesthesia or IV diazepam has been tried).

Contractures, like other less glamorous aspects of disease, must become a multidisciplinary area of concern. Where interest leads to research, more resources and improvements follow.

Key points

- Synovial joints must move to remain healthy.
- Joint immobility affects bone, cartilage, muscle, ligaments and synovium with the development of adhesions and fibro-fatty connective tissue.
- In longstanding cases bone fusion around the joint can occur.
- The common causes of immobility leading to contractures are joint pain, spasticity, fetal posture and burns.
- Joint pain can be reduced by various methods (e.g. drugs, physical means).
- Orthotics (splints) can be used to immobilize joints temporarily to decrease pain or to maintain gains in the range of movement (serial splinting).
- The prevention of spastic contractures depends on good positioning of the patient as well as assisted limb movements.
- Slow sustained traction will reduce tone for several minutes.

FURTHER READING

Johnstone M. *Restoration of Motor Function in the Stroke Patient.* Churchill Livingstone, Edinburgh, 1978.

Lee JM, Warren MP. *Cold Therapy in Rehabilitation.* Bell and Hyman, London, 1978.

Lehmann JF, *et al.* Therapeutic heat and cold. *Clin Orthopaed* 1974: **99**:207–247.

Nickel VL. Physical rehabilitation of the stroke patient with emphasis on the needs for integration into the community. In: *Stroke: Proceedings of the Ninth Pfizer Symposium.* Churchill Livingstone, Edinburgh, 1976.

26 DEPRESSION

- Signs
- Causes of depression
- Pathogenesis
- Occurrence
- Assessment
- Management
- Prognosis for recovery

SIGNS

Depression is common but may be masked by physical symptoms in older people, leading to a missed diagnosis. Typically the patient has characteristic features of a depressed mood, and may be tearful, anxious, and lack concentration. There may also be weight loss, sleep disturbance, and loss of libido. Depression is not a single diagnosis, but comprises several well recognized syndromes: major depression, minor depression, psychotic major depression, seasonal affective disorder, adjustment disorder with depressed mood, organic affective disorder, dysthymia, and bipolar disorders (manic depressive syndromes). Great progress has been made in producing explicit criteria for classifying patients into these diagnostic groups, and the criteria of the *Diagnostic and Statistical Manual* of the American Psychiatric Association are now widely used (see, for example, Table 26.1). The treatment and prognosis of these different types varies, so there is an increasing emphasis on categorizing depression.

Table 26.1 DSM-III criteria of major depressive illness

A. Essential feature: dysphoric mood or loss of interest/pleasure in usual activities

B. Other symptoms: at least four of the following
 1. Appetite or weight change
 2. Sleep difficulty or hypersomnia
 3. Loss of energy, fatiguability or tiredness
 4. Loss of interest or pleasure in usual activities (including sexual drive)
 5. Feeling of self-reproach or inappropriate guilt
 6. Diminished ability to think or concentrate
 7. Recurrent thoughts of death or suicide or suicidal behaviour

C. Duration at least two weeks

D. Exclusions: patients with
 1. Schizophrenic symptoms
 2. Organic mental disorder
 3. Residual-type schizophrenia
 4. Simple bereavement.

In old age, hypochondriasis and importuning behaviour (i.e. persistently attracting the attention of staff with minor problems) may give the clue to an underlying depressive illness. Symptoms more typical of psychotic illness, such as paranoid delusions and hallucinations — particularly of disintegration and smelliness — may occur. Suicide is relatively common amongst elderly depressives, and much more often successful than among younger people, where attempts far outweigh suicides. Depression may be the underlying cause of any of the common presentations of illness in old age: confusion, immobility and falls, incontinence, and inability to cope.

Some elderly patients become severely withdrawn and are at great risk of dying from dehydration and malnutrition. It is vital to recognize their perilous state and ensure that vigorous treatment is given, both to resuscitate and to treat the depression. Often this may entail electroconvulsive therapy (ECT).

Rarely, patients present with non-specific symptoms, and have extensive investigations which find nothing. A trial of antidepressants may result in a dramatic improvement, and a presumptive diagnosis of depression is made.

CAUSES OF DEPRESSION

Life events

Old age may be seen as intrinsically depressing, associated as it is with losses — job, status, abilities, bereavements. There is considerable evidence that major life events are associated with depression at all ages, and particularly in old age. People with supportive social contacts, with a confidante, tend to weather the storm of losses better than those without. It may be that it is not the losses themselves that are significant, but the elderly person's resilience to the changes induced by losses.

Loss of special senses

Loss of hearing and of vision are associated with increased risk of depression. It is likely that the reduced sensory input leads to disengagement, both within the family and the wider world. Over time the lack of social contact and intercourse may make the person less able to cope with changes, more withdrawn, and vulnerable to depression.

Associations with physical illness

Depressive symptoms commonly accompany physical disease, particularly stroke, heart disease, Parkinson's disease and severe arthritis. Often the symptoms are relatively mild, and do not warrant a diagnosis of depressive illness or the use of antidepressant drugs. Control of the underlying physical illness, particularly pain and immobility, may lead to improvement in mood. However, patients who do not improve during rehabilitation may be suffering with depression leading to poor concentration, negative feelings and 'poor motivation'. These patients often do respond well to antidepressants and the importance of diagnosing their symptoms is obvious.

PATHOGENESIS

The underlying biological changes in depression are not fully understood, but there is evidence that catecholamine (adrenaline and noradrenaline) levels in the brain are low. This theory is attractive because catecholamines are responsible for arousal; hence low levels might be expected to lead to depression. Further support comes from the antidepressant effect of drugs that increase the effective amounts of catecholamines in brain nerve endings by reducing the activity of enzymes that destroy catecholamines — the monoamine oxidase inhibitors.

It is likely that the mechanisms of depression are multiple and complex. A more recently researched class of brain messenger 5-hydroxytryptamine (5-HT), also seems to be involved in regulation of mood. Drugs designed to increase 5-HT activity are also potent antidepressants. The precise nature of biological damage that causes depression is still uncertain, but research using radio-isotope labelled neurotransmitters and positron emission tomography to define which parts of the brain and which messengers are active and inactive in depressed patients will help unravel the mystery.

OCCURRENCE

The prevalence of depressive illness is high in old age, and is more common amongst women than men (Table 26.2). In very old people the prevalence falls, suggesting that susceptibility is less in those who have greater survival potential. This may be related to the better social networks which are related to both survival and low risk of depression.

Questionnaire

Your answers to the questions will help us in our research. We are interested in how you are feeling generally and all answers are *entirely confidential*. Some of the questions may seem strange but we would be most grateful if you would answer them anyway. Simply tick the box next to the statement that seems most appropriate for you.

There are 12 questions in all.

1. In general, how is your health compared with others of your age?
   (Please tick one box only)
   ☐ Excellent
   ☐ Good
   ☐ Fair
   ☐ Don't know what is meant by question

2. How quick are you in your physical movements compared with a year ago?
   (Please tick one box only)
   ☐ Quicker than usual
   ☐ About as quick as usual
   ☐ Less quick than usual
   ☐ Considerably slower than usual
   ☐ Don't know what is meant by question

3. How much energy do you have, compared to a year ago?
   (Please tick one box only)
   ☐ More than usual
   ☐ About the same as usual
   ☐ Less than usual
   ☐ Hardly any at all
   ☐ Don't know what is meant by question

4. In the last month, have you had any headaches?
   (Please tick one box only)
   ☐ Not at all
   ☐ About the same as usual
   ☐ Some of the time
   ☐ A lot of the time
   ☐ All of the time
   ☐ Don't know what is meant by question

5. Have you worried about things this past month?
   (Please tick one box only)
   ☐ Not at all
   ☐ Only now and then
   ☐ Some of the time
   ☐ A lot of the time
   ☐ All of the time
   ☐ Don't know what is meant by question

6. Have you been sad, unhappy (depressed) or weepy this past month?
   (Please tick one box only)
   ☐ Not at all
   ☐ Only now and then
   ☐ Some of the time
   ☐ A lot of the time
   ☐ All of the time
   ☐ Don't know what is meant by question

7. In the past month, have you been lying awake at night feeling uneasy or unhappy?
   (Please tick one box only)
   ☐ Not at all
   ☐ Once or twice
   ☐ Quite often
   ☐ Very often
   ☐ Don't know what is meant by question

8. Do you blame yourself for unpleasant things that have happened to you in the past?
   (Please tick on box only)
   ☐ Not at all
   ☐ About one thing
   ☐ About a few things
   ☐ About everything
   ☐ Don't know what is meant by question

9. How do you feel about your future?
   (Please tick one box only)
   ☐ Very happy
   ☐ Quite happy
   ☐ All right
   ☐ Unsure
   ☐ Don't care
   ☐ Worried
   ☐ Frightened
   ☐ Hopeless
   ☐ Don't know what is meant by question

10. What have you enjoyed doing lately?
    (Please tick one box only)
    ☐ Everything
    ☐ Most things
    ☐ Some things
    ☐ One or two things
    ☐ Nothing
    ☐ Don't know what is meant by question

11. In the past month, have there been times when you've felt quite happy?
    (Please tick one box only)
    ☐ Often
    ☐ Sometimes
    ☐ Now and then
    ☐ Never
    ☐ Don't know what is meant by question

12. In general, how happy are you?
    (Please tick one box only)
    ☐ Very happy
    ☐ Fairly happy
    ☐ Not very happy
    ☐ Not happy at all
    ☐ Don't know what is meant by question

Figure 26.1 The Selfcare (D) rating scale for depression (reproduced with permission from Bird *et al.*, 1987)

Table 26.2 Prevalence of depression

| Age group | In the community | | Under Part 3 of the 1948 Act | Long-term care in hospital |
	M	F		
65–74	6.0%	12.0%	16.6%	35%
75+	5.5%	10.5%		

ASSSESSMENT OF DEPRESSION

Depression, though treatable, is frequently missed by doctors and nurses. The problem arises partly because of the altered, more physical presentation of the disease. In addition, there is a tendency to assume that depression is a normal response to the adversity of old age — 'I'd be depressed too if that happened to me'. Increased recognition of the problem is needed, but must be coupled with better management.

Simple self-filled rating scales are available, and give an easy means of picking up people who will require a more thorough assessment. The questions in such scales may usefully be used by doctors and nurses as part of the routine assessment of an elderly patient (Fig. 26.1).

Several of the depression scales do not perform as well with old people as with younger adults. This is because many of them rely on physical markers of depression, that may easily be present in any older person with concurrent physical illness. Such scales tend to produce large numbers of false-positives, people incorrectly labelled as suffering with depression. However, provided it is accepted that simple rating scales are no substitute for proper psychiatric assessment, this should not be a problem since it is better to over-diagnose than to miss such a treatable condition.

Pseudodementia is depressive illness masquerading as dementia. It is easy to see how this happens since the patient may appear confused, lack concentration and perform badly on tests of cognition. Poor self-care and psychomotor retardation combine to give a picture of moderate dementia. Unless thought is given to the possibility of depression, the patient may be inappropriately consigned to long-term institutional care.

Assessment of severity of depression

It is vital that careful assessment for suicidal risk is made so that appropriate management can be given. Severe depression in old people is associated with a high mortality, and admission to hospital is usually necessary so that effective treatment and monitoring may be given. Of great importance in such patients is daily weighing. This gives a good yardstick to monitor both the initial severity (provided that pre-illness weight is known), and response to treatment. Rapid losses in weight are usually due to dehydration and indicate the need for intravenous fluids.

MANAGEMENT

In primary care, even those patients who are diagnosed correctly often receive inappropriate treatment with hypnotics or anxiolytics — the 'Valium (diazepam) syndrome'. However, treating depression is more than simply giving a course of an appropriate antidepressant drug. As in every other aspect of health care of the elderly, an holistic approach is needed.

This is best done by a psychiatry of old age team with direct access to occupational therapy, clinical psychology, and community psychiatric nursing. This will ensure that the patient gets a multidisciplinary assessment, and attention will be given to other physical and social problems that may be aggravating the depressive illness. The general practitioner has a major role in this team as the person who probably knows the patient best, and the person who will be responsible for the continued monitoring of the patient's recovery. Some patients may not wish to be managed by a hospital-based team, particularly in areas where there is substantial stigma to visiting the local psychiatric hospital. In such cases, home visits by a consultant in conjunction with the GP are vital for assessing the severity of the depression, and for ensuring that the patient does get access to services at home. For milder cases of depression, the GP may wish to manage the patient. Provided mood is monitored, and the patient is not experiencing problems with activities of daily living, and if a recurrent problem or previous episodes have been successfully treated, then this obviously saves resources.

Non-specific management

Attention to the small details is of great importance in the overall management of depressed elderly patients. It is crucial that hearing aids and spectacles work, that any underlying pain is adequately relieved, that false teeth are clean and in place, that the patients' self-respect is encouraged by wearing their own clothes, and that dignity is maintained.

The hospital ward environment is often bleak with little source of stimulation besides the television or radio. Use of domestic (rather than institutional) furniture, lighting and paint finishes or wallpaper can help promote a more homely environment. With a little imagination, day rooms can be more like sitting rooms and the rest of the ward more like a series of bedrooms. Emphasizing the identity of patients is necessary, and can be aided by providing space for cherished possessions from home. Many units have managed to obtain the authorization necessary to get a ward cat or dog. Such pets can be a remarkable source of interest and activity among patients recovering from depression.

The patient's day requires more thought than in the acute medical ward setting. Time needs to be given to physical activity that may lead to a faster recovery. Simple ball games, such as throwing a large beach ball around in a circle, may seem childish but help develop psychomotor skills. Mealtimes assume great importance, and are a focal part of the day. The social aspects of eating are used to increase engagement with other patients and staff. Inventiveness is needed to promote activities that engage patients, staff and family, and this is part of the challenge of nursing elderly people.

Many patients will require rehabilitation to resume normal activities of daily living. They need to be given time to practise kitchen skills, getting dressed, and restoring their mobility. Those with longstanding depression may have become physically very weak and stiff, simply through disuse. Active programmes of physiotherapy and occupational therapy are needed for most patients.

Clinical pyschologists are often part of the team, and are extremely helpful in assessing the degree of cognitive impairment of depressed patients, and providing behavioural treatments for patients with phobias, and anxiety states that are associated with depression.

Social work is frequently needed by depressed patients. Often they have given little attention to paying bills or to maintenance of their homes, and have very limited social networks. Advice about finances, about local opportunities for joining clubs, day centres and lunch clubs, and organizing home care services are often of great value in aiding the patient's successful return home.

Psychotherapy for elderly people is such a rarity in the health service, and is quite scarce for those patients able to pay for private care, that its place in the management of depressed elderly patients is unclear. Much of the work of community psychiatric nurses is probably within the sphere of supportive psychotherapy, particularly during the recovery phase.

Antidepressant drugs

Antidepressants are powerful drugs, with potentially serious side-effects (Table 26.3). Care is required in their use, and as with most prescribing in older people, the rule is to start with very low doses and build up slowly. Side-effects are often avoided by using a single night-time dose of drug, and the hypnotic effects of some antidepressants can be useful if sleep disturbance is a problem.

These days, mono-amine oxidase inhibitors (MAOIs) are rarely used as newer antidepressants are both safer and as effective. Occasionally psychiatrists will treat patients with these drugs if response to other drugs has been poor. Tricyclic antidepressants (so called because of the shape of the drug molecule) are most commonly used. Newer versions have fewer anticholinergic side-effects (dry mouth, constipation, postural hypotension, retention of urine, confusional state), but are not completely safe. Careful monitoring of side-effects is still needed. The newest drugs, the 5-HT agonists, seem to have great potential, but experience among elderly patients is quite limited at present.

Lithium is typically used in manic–depressive psychosis, but may be useful as an adjunct in patients who do not respond to tricyclic antidepressants. Side-effects are frequent with lithium, and regular monitoring of serum levels is necessary.

Electroconvulsive therapy has an accepted place in the management of severe depression, and can be very effective in elderly patients, particularly those who are becoming withdrawn and are refusing medication, food and drink. Because of some antipathy to the use of ECT it is sometimes not considered soon enough in patients who are resistant to other forms of treatment.

PROGNOSIS FOR RECOVERY

Depression in old age is not good news, and although the condition is treatable, patients die; up to 14 per cent within a year of diagnosis. However, it is debatable whether death rates are higher than expected, since depressed patients frequently suffer with concurrent life-shortening diseases. Untreated depression may resolve, following a pattern of recurrent episodes. In general the results of treatment are better among older than younger patients. Up to a quarter of treated patients will enjoy a complete recovery within a year of diagnosis, but between a third and a half will still have symptoms.

Table 26.3 Classes of antidepressants and side-effects

	Sedation	Anticholinergic effects	Postural hypotension	Other effects
Tricyclic antidepressants				
Amitriptyline	+++	+++	+++	Heart block
Impipramine	−	+	++	arrhythmias
Nortriptyline	++	++	++	acute glaucoma,
Lofepramine	−	+	++	mania (lofepramine),
Dothiepin	+++	+++	+++	confusion
Mono-amine oxidase inhibitors				
Phenelzine	+	++	+++	Severe reaction with food containing tyramine
5-HT agonists				
Fluoxetine				Flushing, hypotension
Other drugs				
Lithium carbonate	++			Ohyroidfailure, diabetes insipidus toxicity
Carbamazepine				Ataxia, visual disturbance

Little information is available on the continued use of medication after symptoms have disappeared, but drugs are often used for about a year, gently withdrawing treatment. In patients who have suffered relapse routine 'maintenance' therapy is used.

Key points

- Depression is common in old age but may present atypically with non-specific symptoms. It is frequently unrecognized and can be a life-threatening disease.
- Depression is associated with adverse life events (losses), with hearing and visual impairment, and with physical illness.
- Depression can lead to poor performance on tests of cognitive function, suggesting a dementia — this is sometimes termed 'pseudodementia'.
- Management of depression is multidisciplinary, involving the GP, hospital consultant, community psychiatric nurse, clinical psychologist, and occupational therapist, as well as family and other carers.

- Attention to small details is a necessary part of non-specific management.
- Tricyclic antidepressant drugs have serious sidd-effects (anticholinergic: dry mouth, blurred vision, urinary retention, postural hypotension) and low doses must be used initially, building up the dose depending on response.
- Depression in old age has a better prognosis than at younger ages: up to a quarter of patients will get better, but between a third and a half will still have symptoms after a year.

FURTHER READING

Murphy E (ed.). *Affective Illness in the Elderly*. Churchill Livingstone, Edinburgh, 1986.

Wattis J, Hindmarch I (eds). *Psychological Assessment of the Elderly*. Churchill Livingstone, Edinburgh, 1988.

27 PSYCHOTIC AND OTHER DISORDERS

- Hallucinations and delusions
- Paraphrenia
- Management of paranoid symptoms
- Mania
- Schizophrenia
- *Folie à deux*
- Diogenes syndrome
- Jekyll and Hyde syndrome
- Substance abuse

HALLUCINATIONS AND DELUSIONS

Hallucinations are the experience or perception of phenomena that are not present in reality. Delusions are false beliefs that are firmly held despite evidence to the contrary, that are not acceptable or normal within the society or culture, and may be supported by misinterpretations of real phenomena. For example, an hallucination is hearing voices or seeing little people walking around a room, whereas a delusion is believing that a partner is putting poison rather than sugar into the tea.

Hallucinations occurring on falling asleep and on waking are extremely common (hypnogogic and hypnopompic hallucinations) and have no pathological significance at all. However they can be a source of concern to anxious people who may infer that they herald madness.

Hallucinations and delusions are quite common but may be difficult to uncover as patients may be understandably afraid of admitting them, or may include for example the doctor, nurse or carer into a delusional belief system of persecution. A patient's behaviour may be the clue to these symptoms. They may appear frightened, scream or strike out, or start up a conversation without anyone present.

The significance of hallucinations and delusions is much less clear-cut than in younger people. Auditory hallucinations and paranoid delusions are common in severe depressive illness, in mania, and may occur in people with longstanding deafness or visual impairment. Hallucinations also occur in organic brain disease, particularly in alcohol withdrawal (delirium tremens), dementias and after stroke. It is important to realize that medication (particularly L-dopa, opiates, antidepressants, steroids) can cause hallucinations, and to enquire whether this has occurred on prescribing such drugs. The delirium of acute illness may be associated with hallucinations and paranoid delusions, and the psychiatric symptoms may be much more florid than the underlying physical illness.

Hallucinations of the dead partner often occur after bereavement. These can be very vivid, and are often a source of comfort rather than a problem, although some people may fear that madness is not far away and require reassurance that this is normal. Hearing voices and seeing visions might lead some to the belief that the diagnosis is schizophrenia, but first onset of schizophrenia in old age is highly unlikely.

PARAPHRENIA

This term is used to describe a schizophrenia-like illness occurring for the first time in old age. Paranoia is the usual presenting symptom, but unlike chronic schizophrenia, the disease does not lead to deterioration in personality and emotions. The onset is insidious with increasing suspicion that neighbours are interfering with the patient's life. Patients may complain that a neighbour is spreading gossip about them, or is trying to irritate them with noise from the television. Often these delusions become more dramatic with allegations of use of magic rays, tunnelling under the floorboards, use of the television for spying on the patient, and so on.

Sometimes such delusions occur in an isolated person who has always been the sort to 'keep herself to herself', and is frequently considered to be a little eccentric. Despite remarkably strongly held delusions, in a few patients the disease does not progress and the person continues to live a somewhat paranoid life without coming into contact with medical services.

More usually hallucinations develop along with the paranoid delusions and make life intolerable for the sufferer. The hallucinations are usually of voices that are critical of the person, and interfere with thinking and action. It is usually at this stage that help is sought by friends or neighbours because the person's ability to cope with day-to-day life breaks down.

It is essential to decide whether the acute breakdown is due to paraphrenia or to an organic brain syndrome (i.e. delirium from whatever cause, or early dementia). Such patients require careful medical and psychiatric assessment. Frequently underlying acute neurological signs will be found, and the diagnosis of cerebrovascular disease is made. Up to a third of patients with a diagnosis of paraphrenia will develop obvious dementia within a few years, implying that the paranoid symptoms were an early manifestation of organic brain disease.

MANAGEMENT OF PARANOID SYMPTOMS

In general, it is not sensible to reinforce a patient's delusional beliefs or hallucinations; gentle explanation that what is happening is understandable — but not real — is the best line to take. The patient should be nursed in a well-lit room, with the minimum of extraneous noise, and avoidance of frequent changes of position in the ward, and of nursing staff. Hallucinations and delusions caused by organic brain syndromes should be treated by controlling or removing the underlying cause. All patients with these symptoms should be assessed by a psychiatrist who will be able to advise whether the symptoms are part of a depressive illness, a secondary reaction to drugs, acute illness, or due to paraphrenia.

It is usually necessary to treat the symptoms themselves as they can be so distressing. Small doses of major tranquillizers are used: haloperidol or promazine may be useful if agitation is pronounced. Chlorpromazine (Largactil) is not recommended for elderly patients because of its hypotensive effects. Sometimes a hypnotic may be helpful if symptoms are relatively mild. Major tranquillizers may have serious Parkinsonian side-effects and it is essential to monitor the patient's mobility and tone, reducing the dose if side-effects occur. Routine use of anticholinergic drugs (e.g. benzhexol, orphenadrine) in an attempt to prevent Parkinsonism is not recommended because these drugs are potent causes of confusional states and postural hypotension in old age.

The longer-term management of paranoid patients is likely to require psychiatric rehabilitation, re-engagement into usual activities, and social support. Correction of visual and hearing impairment should be given a high priority. The prognosis of paraphrenia is relatively good with over 90 per cent achieving some degree of recovery.

MANIA

Mania is usually encountered as part of a bipolar illness: one pole being depression and the other mania. The patient oscillates between the two, although the manic symptoms may be relatively mild (hypomania) and not lead to medical attention. A past history of episodes of depressive illness is frequent.

Manic patients are usually over-active, over-talkative, and may also have paranoid delusions. They are usually great fun to talk to as the flight of ideas and pressure of speech, together with grandiose ideas, are entertaining. Occasionally the mania will lead to extravagant acts such as spending large sums of money, or destroying the furniture in an effort to redecorate.

Mania can be due to underlying physical illness, usually a stroke or brain tumour, or to medication (tricyclic antidepressants, psychostimulants, anticholinergics). Treatment is then removal of the underlying cause, and use of major tranquillizers to control the manic symptoms. If the mania is part of a bipolar illness, then long-term control with lithium is the usual management.

SCHIZOPHRENIA

Schizophrenia is usually seen in its 'burnt out' form amongst long-term residents of psychiatric hospitals who have reached old age. The disintegration of personality, the loss of emotions, the thought disturbance are usually less apparent, and often it is only the lip-smacking and tongue writhing (tardive dyskinesia) due to treatment with major tranquillizers that sets a schizophrenic patient apart from other residents in a long-stay institution. However, the auditory hallucinations and paranoid ideas may remain and come to the fore from time to time.

FOLIE À DEUX

This is a rare, but rather delightful, sharing of a delusional belief by two people, usually husband and wife. The delusion is usually paranoid in nature and directed towards neighbours who are believed to be hostile to the couple. The delusion is extremely difficult to treat, as the couple reinforce each others beliefs. Fortunately, it is not usually associated with other psychopathology, and the delusions are relatively mild. It is worth being aware of *folie à deux* so that delusions are not inappropriately believed and acted upon by doctors, nurses, police or others.

DIOGENES SYNDROME

Diogenes was a Greek philosopher who took to living in an earthenware jar. By the end of his life the jar had presumably become pretty squalid, and the syndrome refers to people who live in extreme squalor. Typical sufferers are reclusive men, who are often horders of apparently useless material such as newspapers, empty jars and bottles. Usually the person will have held down a job until retirement age, but will have very few social contacts, and will have remained single. Sometimes the syndrome is associated with schizophrenia or alcohol abuse, although the majority are not ill, but simply eccentric. Some patients with paraphrenia may be wrongly suspected of having the Diogenes syndrome if they keep their paranoid delusions and hallucinations to themselves. It is helpful for all these patients to see an experienced psychiatrist who will be able to elicit such symptoms. Cleaning up their homes usually leads to a return to the orginal squalor within a matter of weeks, and is only possible if intercurrent illness has led to their removal from home, as most refuse all forms of help.

JEKYLL AND HYDE SYNDROME

The patient is admitted from home in an acute crisis of immobility, incontinence and acopia (an acute state of inability to cope with life — often applied to carers as well as patients). Once in hospital the patient becomes self-caring within a day or so. No acute illness is found, nor any psychiatric symptoms. All seems well so discharge is arranged. The patient usually returns to hospital in the same state as before within the week; hence the label Jekyll and Hyde syndrome. The prognosis for independent life at home is poor and most patients find themselves in institutional care.

SUBSTANCE ABUSE

Alcohol

Alcohol abuse affects between 5 and 12 per cent of old people, depending on the definitions used. Elderly drinkers fall into two main groups: those who have drunk all their lives and present with the long-term consequences of abuse, and those who start in late life, usually as a result of bereavement. The prognosis for the latter group is much better than for the former.

A high index of suspicion is needed to make the diagnosis of alcohol abuse. Often drinking is an unrecognized cause of falls, hypothermia, or confusion. The management of acute alcohol syndromes (delirium tremens, Wernecke–Korsakoff's syndrome) is the same as at younger ages. It is essential that high doses of thiamine are given to avoid permanent brain damage.

Frequently, longstanding drinkers have evidence of cirrhosis of the liver, unsteadiness on walking (due to degeneration of the cerebellum), and heart failure due to damage to the heart. The life expectation for such people is not good, but both they and their families may gain support from Alcoholics Anonymous.

Tobacco

It is usually felt, by health professionals, that old people should be allowed to enjoy their cigarettes and not be lectured about giving up. Old people are more enlightened, and in surveys a majority of smokers claim to be interested in giving up, and would value help. Main forces for giving up are the example to be set to young grandchildren, and for a minority their own health. Since life expectation has increased so much after retirement age, and the benefits of stopping smoking are apparent within 4–5 years at younger ages, it is reasonable to support giving up smoking in any elderly person with a life expectation of over 10 years. The methods that are effective with younger adults (one-to-one counselling, hypnosis, substitute behaviour) are likely to as useful with elderly people.

```
┌─────────────────┐
│  Key points     │
└─────────────────┘
```

- Delusions and hallucinations may be caused by organic brain disease (dementia, stroke, acute confusional states, delirium tremens), and may be associated with depression.
- Paraphrenia, a schizophrenia-like illness, is quite common and may be due to an underlying dementia. Treatment with major tranquillizers is usually associated with a good prognosis.
- Mania is usually part of a bipolar illness, but can be caused by organic brain syndromes.
- Alcohol abuse is common and often occult. A high index of suspicion is needed, and treatment with thiamine should be started if there is any likelihood of alcohol abuse.

FURTHER READING

Barrios G, Brook P. Visual hallucinations and sensory delusions in the elderly. *Br J Psychiat* 1984; **144**: 662–664.

Isaacs AD, Post F (eds). *Studies in Geriatric Psychiatry.* John Wiley, New York, 1978.

Kafetz K, Cox M. Alcohol excess and the senile squalor syndrome. *J Am Geriatr Soc* 1982; **30**:706.

28 PALLIATIVE CARE

- Recognition
- Hospices
- Living Wills
- Euthanasia
- Good medical practice
- Pain control
- The general practitioner

In most people's minds the words 'palliative care' (which are preferred to 'terminal care') mean the last few days of a person's life, the use of drugs to control pain and an image of separateness, the dying person being outside of and excluded from conventional health care. This image has not arisen recently. Dying and death have remained taboo subjects for many centuries but socio-culturally current generations are legitimately avoiding 'dying' until maturity, many adults only being exposed to the situation when a very elderly parent dies.

RECOGNITION

The diagnosis that a condition is irreversible and will cause the person to die within a definable short period is never easy. Some conditions are more predictable than others, the certainty of death may come within only hours or days of the event. Despite the universal fact that we will all die there has been an awesome failure to understand this event, compared with birth. Cultural and religious views have moulded our attitudes to those of fearful avoidance.

This professional neglect has been realized and slowly the accumulated knowledge base is being disseminated. As health care workers we are becoming aware of the art and skill needed to break and explain bad news, to expect and understand the reactions of disbelief, denial, anger and resentment. We are learning about how different societies react to death. The time scale of caring in this situation is changing for in some disease states we must allow for the process of palliative care to last for years. We have only begun to evaluate the role of psychological approaches, counselling and holistic/alternative medicine.

HOSPICES

The hospice movement has been one impetus towards change with the pioneering work of Cicely

Saunders and others. Hospices, despite their rapid growth, still care for only about 5 per cent of those dying each year. Yet in their teaching role they are exerting a far greater influence — by raising the standards of palliative care of those people dying in hospital or at home. Recently, however, there has been the impact of AIDS in this area (especially in the USA). The fact that death is suddenly confronting a large, articulate and questioning number of younger people in society places the topic of palliative care under critical scrutiny. Unfortunately the subject and whole process has been found to be lacking in many fundamental aspects. The American gay movement has led the way in support and counselling schemes and information networks. They have stressed the important fact that *we live until we die*, and how we live during this time is what matters. The gay movement has also spawned numerous effective pressure groups trying to ensure adequate funding and a high public profile over the issue of dying.

LIVING WILLS

Attitudes are certainly changing. There is a small but increasing interest in information that might help the individual avoid a protracted illness. One such scheme is known as a *Living Will*. This refers to a document whereby a person while still mentally competent specifies the health care he wishes to receive should he ever become mentally incompetent owing to brain damage or dementia. Such a document has no legal validity in the UK but has been adopted by most of the States in the USA. In addition to the Living Will an enduring power of attorney (for health care) allows the competent person to appoint an advocate to act on their behalf and act as the 'fine tuning' to the whole mechanism. The belief is that the Living Will returns autonomy to an otherwise disenfranchised adult and is a departure from a very paternalistic area of medicine.

Views in this area run along a spectrum — from the concept of it being morally wrong, through the premise that good medical practice already allows people to die in certain circumstances, to the notion that this form of legislation (if adopted) falls short of the ultimate upholding of autonomy and dignity, that is the right to die at a time of one's own choosing (i.e. euthanasia). Living Wills (generically called advance directives) are usually in a prescribed form of declaration, but can vary as to complexity. An example is given below.

1. If the time comes when I am incapacitated to the point when I can no longer actively take part in decisions for my own life, and am unable to direct my physician as to my own medical care, I request that I be allowed to die and not be kept alive through life-sustaining measures if my condition is deemed irreversible. I do not intend any direct taking of my life, but only that my dying not be unreasonably prolonged.

2. It is my express wish that if I should develop

   (a) brain disease of severe degree; or
   (b) serious brain damage resulting from accidental or other injury or illness, or
   (c) advanced malignant disease, in which I would be unable or mentally incompetent to express my own opinion about accepting or declining treatment;

   and if two independent physicians conclude that, to the best of current medical knowledge, my condition is irreversible, then I request that the following points (3)–(6) be taken into consideration.

3. Any separate illness (e.g. pneumonia, or a cardiac or kidney condition) which may threaten my life should not be given active treatment unless it appears to be causing me undue physical suffering. Cardiopulmonary resuscitation should not be used if the existing quality of my life is already seriously impaired.

4. In the course of such an advanced illness, if I should be unable to take food, fluid or medication, I would wish that these should not be given by any artificial means, except for the relief of obvious suffering.

5. If, during any such an illness, my condition deteriorates and, as a result, my behaviour becomes violent, noisy, or in any other ways degrading, or if I appear to be suffering severe pain, any symptom should be controlled immediately by appropriate drug treatment, regardless of the consequences upon my physical health and survival, to the extent allowed by law.

6. The object of this declaration is to minimise distress or indignity which I may suffer or create during an incurable illness, and to spare my medical advisers and/or relatives the burden of making difficult decisions on my behalf.

EUTHANASIA

An even more controversial area of debate surrounds the subject of euthanasia — the deliberate taking of life. This has aroused much interest recently, with the Netherlands not legalizing the issue but under clearly set out guidelines not prosecuting the doctors involved in carrying out euthanasia. The criteria are quite strict (competence issues, certainty of near death, etc.), but the doctors taking part certainly see it as an extension of their caring role — indeed caring up to and including death. The client chooses the time and place and sleep is induced by an intravenous drug and death occurs by the same route (potassium chloride is used). The procedure is explained beforehand and verbal refusal at any stage cancels the 'agreement'. This subject needs to be debated away from the glare of publicity and, together with advance directives, placed in a correct perspective.

GOOD MEDICAL PRACTICE

It is stated that there is an interest in both euthanasia and advance directives because current medical practice is deficient in certain key areas and hence these options are seen as desirable. In the care of the terminally ill,those who are chronically disabled and those with dementia of severe degree, it is important to ask and attempt to define what constitutes good medical practice. Many of these people are elderly. There are no clearly defined guidelines apart from what is permissible by law and many people are unhappy at certain aspects concerning the care of these groups in both institutional and community settings. In the case of long-stay and terminally ill patients, nurses have more frequent, prolonged and personal contact with patients and relatives than have the medical team, and so the opinions of the nursing staff are vitally important in assessing the medical and ethical problems of patient care. The management of a clinical dilemma which involves ethical considerations should be decided upon by a process of open communication between the patient (where possible), doctors, nurses, relatives and other carers and important conclusions should be recorded in the case notes.

The notion of 'quality of life' is essential in this process of assessment and decision making. It is an elusive concept, but various attempts have been made to define it. In the context of the frail elderly, Denham feels that measures of quality of life must include health (mortality and survival), health perception, function and mental health. He also stresses the importance of the quality of the environment. Fear of growing old with physical and mental frailty is usually accompanied by an image of slovenly and dirty clothes, uncontrolled incontinence, disruptive behaviour, or a dulled 'twilight' life of drug-induced stupor in a Victorian workhouse setting. This image is uncomfortable because it has an unpleasantly realistic basis. What can and does happen where imagination and resources are combined is a very different picture.

In the areas of intensive care and cardio-pulmonary resuscitation on patients with terminal malignant disease and dementia, several attempts have been made to develop valid systems for quantifying jointly the stage of the disease, its prognosis, and the burdens on the individual in such a way as to allow an objective evaluation of the quality of life. Well-designed studies have an important place in setting standards.

The science of symptom relief and the art of nursing care are integral and well matched. Dying should occur in the absence of distressing symptoms and distressed patients. However, research shows that relatives are highly critical of the care given in the last stage of a person's life.

This brief summary only focuses on particular areas. It is meant to be a guide and stimulus to further reading and to illustrate that it is ignorance that leads to health care professionals dealing badly with the dying — reinforcing prejudices and fear in the lay public.

PAIN CONTROL

Pain can be a significant problem in advanced cancer yet the majority of patients can be relieved of it without specialist intervention. It is argued that there is often hesitancy to ensure adequate pain relief because of the fear of being seen to hasten the end of life. The goal is full pain relief, no breakthrough pain and as few side-effects as possible. Only in the later stages should dosages impinge on consciousness, and then the relief of pain is part of the dying process not the cause of it. However, it is not only a matter of analgesia: pain is an emotion altered by fear, weakness, and tiredness — hence the broad approach needed.

Patients often have more than one pain and the management is a detailed affair. For each pain, the history and severity should be ascertained and a diagnosis made. The history should include responses to previous treatments. See Table 28.1 for a general plan of treatment.

Table 29.1 Treatment of pain

General
The affective component of pain

Specific (for each pain)
Adequate dose of analgesic for the individual patient
Continuous pain needs continuous medication
Co-analgesics as necessary
Consider non-drug treatments

Objectives (discussed with the patient)
Pain free at night
Pain free at rest
Pain free on movement

Monitor
Review progress soon and often

Analgesics

The following is a general guide:

Mild pain: paracetamol or aspirin
Moderate: weak opioid (dextropropoxyphene)
Severe: morphine

With morphine most patients need a 4-hourly regimen. Doses should start low (2.5–5 mg 4-hourly) and be increased as necessary; some patients eventually need more than 30 mg 4-hourly. Elderly and frail patients should always be started on the smaller doses and the response assessed. Pain relief is the aim, and not a fast route to unconsciousness. Using an aqueous solution of morphine the dosage can be increased without increase in the volume of liquid taken. For many patients a controlled release preparation of morphine (MST) is available in tablet form in various dosages. Rectal administration of drugs (morphine and oxycodone suppositories) can be used if a patient is unable to take oral drugs. In some cases prolonged parenteral administration is needed and a syringe pump is used. The side-effects of opioids (constipation, nausea and vomiting) are amenable to treatment if they occur. Indeed, constipation is so common that laxatives should be given routinely.

Co-analgesics

These are drugs or devices which may not have intrinsic pain relieving activity but when used with conventional analgesics will aid pain relief. Examples are diazepam, psychotropics, corticosteroids, and muscle relaxants.

Non-drug measures

Flowtron (a pneumatic compression sleeve) for lymphoedema, radiotherapy, chemotherapy and hormone treatments, palliative surgery, nerve blocks, neurosurgery, massage, relaxation hypnotherapy, acupuncture, diet, transcutaneous nerve stimulation and biofeedback techniques may all have a place in management. The multiplicity of methods suggests that specialist help is needed in guiding choice of management in those not helped by single treatments. Other major symptoms of the terminally ill can be assessed and treated similarly. Cough can be suppressed, dyspnoea (shortness of breath) relieved, nausea and vomiting controlled. Weakness and confusion are perhaps harder to treat. Confusion can result from polypharmacy, comparatively minor intercurrent infections and other causes which, when found and treated, may reverse some of the confusion. The art of nursing the terminally ill requires communication, listening and responding to anxieties. It involves helping to maintain dignity and some independence until death. Prevention of other complications such as pressure sores by adequate support mechanisms is essential. When mobility is limited (as in weakness) a wheelchair is a useful adjunct. Continence aids sometimes require expert assistance from the continence adviser. Catheters/penile sheaths can make a patient comfortable and less exhausted, while leg bags mean that dignity is maintained.

THE GENERAL PRACTITIONER

The GP is the resource centre both practically and often emotionally to the patient and the family. The GP often makes the diagnosis or is involved on discharge from hospital. The GP also acts as the 'key worker' to all the primary health care services, the Social Services as well as specialist groups such as psychiatrists (in the treatment of depression), bereavement counselling, home terminal care schemes, pain relief clinics, in-patient hospice care, etc. Other support groups are often part of this network: neighbours, friends, church and self-help groups.

| Key points |

- Many people do not experience the death of a close relative until reaching mature adulthood.
- Hospices only care for about 5 per cent of those dying each year.
- Death and dying are still taboo subjects surrounded by myth and ignorance, but the impact of AIDS is changing the way the subject of palliative care is being addressed.
- Living Wills (generically called advance directives) are statements of wish with reference to health care in the case of the subject becoming mentally incompetent.
- Livings Wills plus an enduring power of attorney (for health issues) are valid in the USA, allow some autonomy of an incompetent patient's wishes and are the subject of intense debate.
- Euthanasia is an entirely separate issue from Living Wills. It is the deliberate taking of life. Controlled access is available to people in the Netherlands where some doctors view it as an extension of their caring role. Strict guidelines are enforced there and euthanasia can only be carried out on mentally competent individuals.
- Measures of quality of life include health (mortality and survival), health perception, function, mental health and the quality of the environment.
- The science of symptom relief and the art of nursing care are integral and well matched.

- In pain control the goal is full pain relief, no breakthrough pain and as few side-effects as possible.
- Assessment of pain includes identifying individual pains with a *pain chart*.
- Treatment which results in the subject being continuously pain-free will involve dose monitoring and the use of various analgesics, co-analgesics and non-drug measures.
- The GP is the key worker in terminal/palliative care at home.

FURTHER READING

Age Concern. *Living Wills: Consent to Treatment at the End of Life.* Age Concern Working Party Report, Edward Arnold, London, 1988.

Denham M. Assessment of quality of life. In: *Care of Long-Stay Elderly Patients.* Croom Helm, Beckenham, 1983.

Kubler-Ross E. *On Death and Dying.* Tavistock, London, 1970.

Parkes CM. *Bereavement: Studies of Grief in Adult Life.* Penguin, Harmondsworth, 1980.

Rachels J. *The End of Life (Euthanasia and Morality).* Oxford University Press, London, 1986.

Saunders C. A therapeutic community: St Christopher's Hospice. In: *Psychological Aspects of Terminal Care.* Columbia University Press, 1972.

Update Postgraduate Centre. *Terminal Care.* Update Siebert Publications, 1986.

29 BETTER PRESCRIBING

- Adverse drug reactions
- Reasons for adverse reactions
- Compliance

Elderly people are frequent users of prescribed medication. Over the years, they are the only age group that has had an increase in the amount of medication prescribed. In 1977 the average pensioner received about 11 prescription drugs a year, but by 1985 this had risen to about 15 drugs a year, almost three times the national average. This increased prescribing for older people arises in part because they suffer with multiple diseases which need treatment, and in part because doctors tend to respond to every symptom by prescribing a medication. The common drugs used in the old age group are more often prescribed the older people get, certainly up to the age of 80 years (see Fig. 29.1).

It is debatable whether so many elderly patients really require treatment with diuretics, benzodiazepines, and non-steroidal anti-inflammatory pain killers.

ADVERSE DRUG REACTIONS

If drugs were free of side-effects then it might not matter too much, but all the commonly used drugs can have major adverse effects. Measuring the occurrence of adverse drug reactions is complicated, because of the wide range of different drugs used, the different durations of use, and the range of adverse effects which may be trivial or life-threatening. Consequently many studies of adverse drug reactions report data that are difficult to interpret.

All the evidence points to older people being at greater risk of adverse reactions. For example, fatal reactions occur about four times more often in patients over 70 than at younger ages. Adverse effects of hypnotics are more common in older patients, even at low doses.

REASONS FOR ADVERSE REACTIONS

Inadequate clinical assessment

The greatest danger to the patient is the knee-jerk response doctor: joint pain equals non-steroidal anti-inflammatory pain killer; ankle oedema equals diuretic. Poor assessment of the need for therapy is a major preventable cause of adverse reactions.

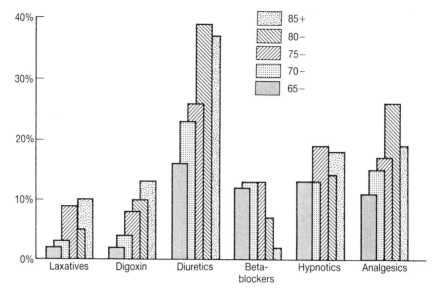

Figure 29.1 Variations in drug use with age (Cartright and Smith, 1988)

Excessive prescribing

Both the dose of drug and the number of drugs used are related to risk of adverse effects. A general principle with elderly patients is to start with the lowest possible dose and work up gradually. This is, of course, time-consuming but is essential for safe prescribing. A case where elderly patients differ is the use of L-dopa preparations (Sinemet, Madopar) in Parkinson's disease, where some neurologists will start patients on large doses to demonstrate an effect and then work the dose downwards. Another example is the use of antidepressant drugs which are often given in very high dose in younger patients, but are usually effective in much lower doses in old age.

The number of drugs given should be tempered by a sense of what is reasonable. Treatment schedules, particularly in hospital, seem quite unreasonable, with many different medications prescribed. It is useful to set priorities and aim to examine the effects of treating a single problem, rather than treating every disease process simultaneously. Many patients avoid excessive prescribing by simply not taking all their medications!

Inadequate supervision of long-term medication

Beware of the repeat prescription. In many general practices it is usual to insist that repeat prescriptions are only issued without review for a fixed time, say six months. Further problems can arise when different doctors treat the patient and are not aware of existing medications; this can happen easily when patients attend clinics and day hospitals. It is wise to have a policy that all prescribing is done by one doctor, usually the general practitioner.

Altered pharmacokinetics and pharmacodynamics (Table 29.1)

These aspects of prescribing in old age usually receive far too much emphasis, as most of the age-related changes in drug handling (with the exception of reduced renal excretion — see below) are not very important. Very limited information is available about pharmacodynamic changes (i.e. in receptor sensitivity to drug molecules) with age. However, elderly people appear to have a greater sensitivity to the effects of benzodiazepines, and perform tasks less well at a given dose than younger subjects. By contrast, beta-blocker drugs are less effective in old age. This may be because elderly people have fewer active receptor sites for the drug molecules to occupy.

The *absorption of drugs* is generally unchanged in elderly people, with the exception of drugs that are metabolized to active compounds by the liver (e.g. major tranquillizers and tricyclic antidepressants). In such cases, the absorption of the drug is greater than expected, leading to a greater bioavailability and greater effect; hence the usual advice to give small doses of drugs to elderly patients.

Table 29.1 Changes in pharmacokinetics

Drug absorption
Unchanged

Drug distribution
Increase in distribution volume of lipid(fat)-soluble drugs
Decrease in distribution volume of water-soluble drugs

Hepatic metabolism
Reduced liver mass
Reduced phase-I pathways

Renal excretion
Decreased glomerular filtration rate and tubular secretion

The *volume of distribution* of a drug depends on whether it is water-soluble or lipid (fat)-soluble. With age, the ratio of fat to lean muscle increases, leading to fat-soluble drugs having more space to spread around, thus exerting their effects for a longer time. For example, benzodiazepines have a prolonged elimination time, leading to prolonged effects, because they are fat-soluble and more widely distributed. Water-soluble drugs tend to have a smaller volume of distribution, leading to rapid peak effects following a dose. Examples include alcohol, digoxin and cimetidine. None of these effects has great clinical significance beyond the golden rule of low doses for old people.

Liver metabolism involves the oxidation, reduction and hydrolysis (phase-I pathways) and glucuronidation, acetylation, and sulfation (phase-II pathways) of drugs. The phase-I pathways tend to be reduced in old age, leading to reduced elimination of some drugs, such as benzodiazepines.

Reduction in renal excretion is an important aspect of pharmacokinetics. Many drugs are excreted in urine, and reduced glomerular filtration and tubular secretion can lead to serious accumulation. The best examples are aminoglycoside antibiotics, lithium, chlorpropramide and digoxin, all of which can build up to dangerous levels.

COMPLIANCE

It is traditional to blame the patient for poor compliance — for not doing what the doctor says. However, several factors can lead to poor compliance. The patient must know why the medication is needed and should understand the expected effects and the instructions for use. Doctors seldom spend sufficient time explaining, and make limited use of tablet cards and drug information leaflets to aid understanding and medicine taking (see Table 29.2).

There is a wide range of pill holders that can be of some help in reminding patients when to take their medication and, as importantly, what they need to take (see Fig. 29.2). In general, the simplest devices are the most useful. They consist of a plastic box for each day of the week, divided into morning, lunchtime and evening. A relative, or the patient, places the correct drugs for the week in the correct positions. However, the patient must be sensible enough to remember that they need to take medication.

Table 29.2 Rules of prescribing

1. Make a careful clinical assessment
2. Know your drugs: side effects, doses
3. Use low starting doses
4. Simplify dose and drug regime
5. Review the medication regularly
6. Maintain good compliance: check for problems
7. Communicate with general practitioner, patient and family
8. Remember about adverse drug reactions: notify all of them
9. When in doubt, don't prescribe.

Figure 29.2 Boxes to aid compliance

Labelling of bottles, and the type of container, can give elderly patients problems. The increasingly

Table 29.3 Aids to better compliance

1. Explain why the drug is needed
2. Give information about the drug's effects and side-effects
3. Make use of tablet cards and pill holders
4. Label bottles with clear instructions in large type
5. Avoid blister packs and child-proof containers
6. Review medication at each encounter

popular 'blister' packs can be extremely difficult for arthritic fingers to open. It is always worth looking at medication with the patient so that both you and the patient can see what is being given, and go over the reasons for the prescription (see Table 29.3).

Always remember that the prime function of a doctor is to treat the patient and not his own anxieties: 'I feel that when my doctor writes me a prescription for Valium, its to put *him* out of my misery!'

Key points

- Up to 80 per cent of women over 75 years are on at least one prescribed medication. Much treatment with diuretics, benzodiazepines and non-steroidal anti-inflammatory drugs is unnecessary.
- Adverse drug reactions increase in frequency in old age. Adverse reactions and unnecessary prescribing can be avoided by improved clinical assessment, using low drug doses, reducing the number of medications, and by regular review of patients on long-term medication.

- The most important change in pharmacodynamics is reduced renal excretion of drugs such as digoxin, aminoglycoside antibiotics, oral hypoglycaemics and lithium.
- Compliance with medication can be improved by careful explanation of reasons for treatment, expected drug effects and side-effects, use of tablet cards, pill holders, and by better labelling of bottles.
- If in doubt, don't write a prescription!

FURTHER READING

Cartwright A, Smith C. *Elderly People, their Medicines and their Doctors*. Routledge, London, 1988.

30 ELDER ABUSE AND INADEQUATE CARE

- Definitions
- The abused and the abuser
- Recognition
- Social assessment
- Management and intervention
- Prevention and legislation

DEFINITIONS

The 1980s saw the recognition of the phenomenon of elder abuse. Eastman defines it as 'the physical, emotional and psychological abuse of an older person by a formal or informal carer. The abuse is repeated and is the violation of a person's human and civil rights by a person or persons who have power over the life of a dependent'.

Eight major categories of abuse have been identified (see Table 30.1).

Table 30.1 Major categories of abuse

1. Physical/assault
2. Emotional and verbal abuse (psychological)
3. Financial
4. Deprivation of nutrition
5. Involuntary isolation and confinement
6. Sexual abuse
7. Administration of inappropriate drugs or deprivation of prescribed drugs
8. Deprivation of help in performing activities of daily living

Research in this field (mainly in the USA) is now widening the scope of the debate and some people feel that the previous definitions have been limiting and stigmatizing. Professionals especially have been reluctant to report suspected cases. Fulmer and O'Malley feel that cases of abuse and neglect can be better described as *inadequate care*, defined as the presence of unmet needs for personal care. The needs include all basic requirements as well as those of supportive relationships, the opportunity to define an acceptable lifestyle and the freedom from all forms of violence. Thus elder abuse can be defined as 'the actions of a caretaker that create unmet needs for the elderly person'. Neglect is defined as 'the failure of an individual responsible for caretaking to respond adequately to established needs for care'. It is easier to agree on what is adequate or inadequate care than what is acceptable or unacceptable behaviour.

THE ABUSED AND THE ABUSER

Much attention has been placed on the characteristics of the victim (see Table 30.2). Research on abusers indicates that they tend to be sons, with psychological abuse predominating followed by physical abuse. The abusers were likely to be dependent on the victims for finances, led stressful lives and had health and financial problems. One-third had psychological difficulties and even more a history of mental illness and alcohol abuse. It needs to be stated, however, that there is considerable debate surrounding this issue. One school of thought advocates that anyone is a potential abuser if inflicted with sufficient stress. Others feel that abuse is much more likely from individuals with a long history of sociopathic behaviour involved in a caring role, emotionally let alone practically unable to cope.

Table 30.2 Victim characteristics

Elderly over the age of 75
Female
Roleless
Functionally impaired
Lonely
Fearful
Living at home with an adult son or daughter
In addition the person is often heavily immobile,
  incontinent, with negative personality traits

Factors leading to the identification of abuse/inadequate care have been defined (see Table 30.3).

Table 30.3 Factors in identification (after Eastman)

Physical and mental dependence on a key family member
Poor or breakdown of communication
Marked change in carer's lifestyle
Poor perception by carer towards dependence of the older
  person
Frequent visits to GPs by carers to talk about their problems
Role reversal
History of falls and minor injuries
Triggering behaviour: incident that acts as a catalyst inducing loss of control
Cramped or substandard living conditions
Isolation of the household

Other risk factors include people with chronic progressive disabling illnesses (e.g. dementia syndromes, severe arthritis, Parkinson's disease, stroke) that impair function and create care needs that exceed the carer's ability to meet them.

RECOGNITION

This can be extremely difficult because some ageing processes can cause changes which are hard to distinguish from aspects of physical assault (skin bruising can occur easily in the elderly as a result of blood vessels becoming very fragile). Fulmer and

O'Malley's outline of manifestations of inadequate care are shown in Table 30.4.

Table 30.4 Manifestations of inadequate care

Abrasions	Dehydration
Lacerations	Malnutrition
Contusions	Inappropriate clothing
Burns	Poor hygiene
Freezing	Oversedation
Depression	Over/under medication
Fractures	Untreated medical problems
Sprains	Dangerous behaviour
Dislocations	Failure to meet legal
Pressure sores	obligations

Indications of physical violence can include bruises (see Figs. 30.1 and 30.2), welts and fractures. This occurring in the genital area accompanied by vaginal or rectal bleeding (with or without venereal disease) may indicate sexual abuse.

The presence, however, of one or more items from the list of manifestations of inadequate care in Table 30.4 obviously does not establish a diagnosis of abuse or neglect, since the same findings can occur in ill frail elderly people as part of a chronic disease process. In spite of this the presence of these signs should alert the attending doctor to the *possibility* of inadequate care. The most common presentations usually involve combinations of features: poor hygiene, poor nutrition, inadequately managed medical problems, frequent falls, and confusion. Thus the GP, district nurse, health visitor and casualty officer will often be the first people to be presented with the diagnostic dilemmas. Less commonly, legal, Social Services or the police are the agencies first involved because of financial or housing problems.

SOCIAL ASSESSMENT

This aspect may require many interviews over a period of time and can be extremely time-consuming.

Figure 30.1 Skin bruising due to physical assault

Figure 30.2 Skin marks due to restraint

As much information as possible should be obtained, including financial details. Asking the client and carer about a typical day involving all aspects of daily living, as well as about any recent crises, may be very revealing. The person's current mental status is very important, because the most difficult situations involve clients with memory loss. The most sensitive area of questioning is that of actual abusive episodes, detailing verbal and physical incidents. Interviewing the carer is an emotionally difficult situation.

Formal protocols (screening instruments) for use in suspected cases of elder abuse are being developed in the USA. They can be very lengthy to complete but are thorough and likely to provide conclusive information. Currently the only way this important information can be disseminated and an exchange of views obtained in the UK context is at a *case conference* — the mainstay of multidisciplinary exchange.

MANAGEMENT AND INTERVENTION

Access to an elderly person who is receiving inadequate care can be very difficult. Access can mean both the physical as well as the more psychological barriers that people put up around themselves. Three clearly defined groups are the elderly living alone, the elderly in institutions, and the elderly living with the family/carer.

Those living alone may not cooperate through fear of losing all independence, embarrassment or simple stigma or distrust. Clients who are cognitively impaired may need evaluating by a range of professionals. The complex issues of the elderly living with family involve not only the elderly person concerned but the carer. One approach is to focus first on the needs of the carer. A non-judgemental approach implying an acknowledgement of an ongoing difficult job may then allow the needs of the elderly person to be identified.

The elderly in institutions should in theory be less of a problem in that all institutions (be they continuing care wards, old people's homes, private residential or nursing homes) should have regular visits by the statutory authorities. However, numerous reports document the scale and range of institutional abuse.

PREVENTION AND LEGISLATION

In order to develop and use prevention strategies it is useful to summarize some of the current theories/hypotheses concerning abuse.

Theories

Impairment of the older person. The presence of physical and mental impairment makes the older person dependent and hence vulnerable.

Psychopathology of the abuser. Abusers often have personality defects or disorders.

Transgenerational violence. Children (often abused themselves) observe adult violent behaviour in the family and internalize it as acceptable. This can lead to spouse abuse and child abuse and later eventually to parental abuse.

Stressed carer. Carers, especially if subject to their own life crises, react to the stressful situation and dependent person with violence or inadequate care.

Exchange theory. The abuser will continue to abuse as long as he or she gains from it. When the 'exchange' becomes unfavourable (guilt, professional 'knowing', etc.) the abuse ceases.

Discussion

Prevention of inadequate care involves analysing our

current patterns of health and social care delivery. Issues such as housing, pensions, payments for a family carer, and voluntary initiatives are raised. If inadequate care results from impairment of an elderly person or a stressed caregiver, then health and Social Services should be mobilized to try to help both parties. If the carer is psychologically or psychiatrically disturbed then the prevention strategy must protect the client as well as seek trained help for the carer.

The US experience has been to endorse the legal route vigorously. Many States have passed mandatory reporting laws for elder abuse. This has led to the setting up of teams of social workers (Adult Protective Services) to deal with the cases. Health care professionals who fail to report cases can be subject to fines or rebuke from their professional organizations. In the UK, Age Concern favours the setting up of a Charter of Rights to protect the needs of all elderly people.

Whatever the motivating force for change, change must occur. Elder abuse/inadequate care is another iceberg phenomenon. The elderly have an absolute right to expect to be protected from poor care by every means at our disposal. This will need education, research, reallocation of resources and perhaps legislation. Ignoring the problem will not make it go away. Facing it and using expertise developed elsewhere is a positive way forward.

Key points

- There are many types of abuse, but all can be described as inadequate care defined as the presence of unmet needs for personal care.
- The typical victim is an elderly woman, functionally impaired and living at home with an adult son, daughter or husband.
- USA research on abusers indicates that they tend to be sons with psychological/emotional abuse predominating. Abusers were dependent on victims for finances, led stressful lives and had health (especially alcohol and psychological difficulties) and financial problems.
- Risk factors include chronic progressive disabling illnesses, breakdown of communication, isolated or substandard living conditions.

- Factors in identification include frequent visits to GPs by carers with their problems, marked changes in a carer's lifestyle inducing extra stress, and the poor perception by a carer towards the dependence of the older person.
- Recognition of cases is made difficult by the physiological and pathological changes that can occur with ageing (e.g. senile purpura).
- The presence of some of the usual manifestations of inadequate care (abrasions, pressure sores, malnutrition) should alert to the *possibility* of the condition.
- Assessment includes not only a physical examination but a full social history including a sympathetic questioning of the carer's role. The client's mental state must be assessed and recorded.
- A diagnosis of suspected inadequate care must not be made hastily; expert help and advice (social worker, psychiatrist, clincial psychologist) may be necessary.
- Aetiological theories are: impairment of the older person, psychopathology of the abuser, transgenerational violence, stressed carer, and exchange theory.
- The US response to the problem has included legislation (mandatory reporting laws) and a separate social service division (adult protective services).

FURTHER READING

Eastman M. *Old Age Abuse.* Grosvenor Press (Age Concern), Portsmouth, 1984.

Fulmer TT, O'Malley TA. *Inadequate Care of the Elderly.* Springer, New York, 1987.

Kosberg J. Understanding elder abuse: an overview for primary care physicians.In: Ham (ed.), *Geriatric Medicine Annual.* Medical Economics Co., Oradille, NJ, 1987.

Tomlinson S. *Abuse of Elderly People: An Unnecessary and Preventable Problem.* Public Information Report, British Geriatrics Society, London, 1989.

Wolf RS, Pillemer KA. *Helping Elderly Victims: The Reality of Elder Abuse.* Columbia University Press, New York, 1989.

31 ETHNIC ELDERS

- A brief history of migration
- Demography
- Health and social needs
- Ethnic myths
- Providing sensitive services
- A checklist for ethnic elders

Many countries are now home to people who were not born there, and are growing old in a second homeland. Each country has its own unique pattern of migration and links with other countries. Britain is a good example of a multicultural society representing people from many different parts of the world. Many of these people have settled in Britain and consider themselves to be British. Some, particularly more recent arrivals such as Vietnamese and Bangladeshi, although living in Britain, do not identify strongly with British culture. A unifying factor is that all ethnic minorities have contributed and continue to contribute to the economic wealth of the country. The majority pay their taxes and are increasingly concerned by the white ethnocentric bias in the services that they are paying for.

A BRIEF HISTORY OF MIGRATION

The first major movements of 'visible' (i.e. black and Asian) migrants to the UK occurred shortly after the Second World War. Active recruitment policies were used to bring labour from the Caribbean and from India to help with rebuilding postwar Britain. Many of these migrants held the belief that they would be returning to their home countries and the stay in Britain would be but a short sojourn, and an opportunity to accumulate some wealth. These migrants have mostly given up this dream, and once their families followed, they became residents.

These early migrants are now ageing, and many are of pensionable age. Because of recruitment practices, many of them lied about their true ages, claiming to be up to 10 or 15 years younger. Consequently, many men of pensionable age are unable to claim their pensions because of their younger 'passport' age.

During the mid-1970s two further waves of migration occurred: one from East Africa, particularly from Uganda (associated with the Idi Amin regime of terror), of East African Asians, and another from a newly independent country, Bangladesh (formerly East Pakistan). The two groups of migrants could not have been more different. Most of the East African

Asians were originally from Gujarat region of India (around Bombay), and were a sophisticated, well-educated class of merchants and professional people. The Bangladeshi migrants had mostly left because of religious civil war between Hindu and Moslem, and were from the rural areas of Sylhet. Most were landless farmers with little formal education and virtually no money.

Their fortunes in Britain have been shaped by these origins. The East African Asians have found a secure niche in British society, often running corner shops, or returning to professional occupations. The Bangladeshi are concentrated in inner-city slums, particularly in the East End of London, occupying the traditional migrant territory that used to belong to a former generation of Jewish people. Unemployment is high, and opportunities are to be found only in the catering and clothing manufacture industries.

It is important to remember that there are many ethnic minorities in Britain: for example, Irish, Eastern European, Mediterranean, and white South African. Some of the considerations that apply to visible groups may apply to an extent to those minorities that are able to 'blend into' the host culture.

DEMOGRAPHY

Black and Asian people make up less than 4 per cent of the total population of Britain, numbering some 2.5 million people. Yet as an island race, Britons display remarkable xenophobia, feeling overrun by hoards of foreigners. Because of the patterns of migration, the density of minority groups in some parts of the inner-cities turns them into the ethnic majority.

The numbers of pensioners are still comparatively small (see Fig. 31.1). A city the size of Nottingham (population around 400 000) had only 300 Asian and 300 Afro-Caribbean pensioners according to the 1981 census. However, all that is set to change quite rapidly. Most ethnic pensioner groups are going to increase by between two-fold and seven-fold over the next 20 years.

HEALTH AND SOCIAL NEEDS

Traditionally Britain has adopted a policy of assimilation to cope with the needs of ethnic minorities. This means that with time the minorities will adapt to British ways and customs and no special services will

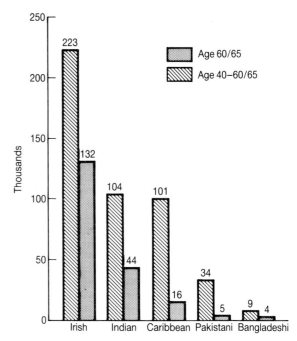

Figure 31.1 Number of ethnic elders according to the 1981 census

be needed. This is a wonderful way of avoiding having any real policy at all! In Canada, assimilation was never an option for the Francophone and Anglophone populations — each was too big to be a 'minority'. Canada has adopted a policy of respecting differences and has set up residential homes that are linguistically and culturally appropriate for most of the minorities living there.

Table 31.1 Health problems of ethnic elders

Tuberculosis
Diabetes
Ischaemic heart disease
Asthma
Stroke
Cataract

In practice, those who work in inner-city areas are already confronted by the lack of suitable services for black and Asian elderly patients. Very few hospitals have a reliable interpreter service, and few hospitals and general practices go out of their way to recruit staff from ethnic minority groups. Consequently it is difficult for patients to get access to services, and even when they do, the standards of practice are likely to be poor because of poor communication and inappropriate or unavailable services.

The major health problems of black and Asian elders are shown in Table 31.1. Although ethnic minorities do suffer with 'exotic' diseases such as sickle cell anaemia, and tropical infections, the greatest burden of disease is caused by common conditions: heart attacks, strokes, diabetes, cataracts. This suggests that the health and social needs should be similar to those of the host community.

However, sick black and Asian elders face serious problems in getting the services they need. The problems have been described as a series of *jeopardies*. The first jeopardy is to do with being a visible ethnic minority — racial prejudice; the second is to do with being old — ageism; and the third is caused by limited access to services.

For example, for a white stroke victim it is possible to arrange a day centre, meals on wheels, a home help, a stroke club. For a Bangladeshi stroke victim there are no day centres, no attempt is made to provide Halal food (meat slaughtered according to Moslem requirements), and stroke clubs do not cater for Bangladeshi people because none of the staff speaks the language. The Bangladeshi patient may be so frail that a residential home is needed, but most boroughs have decided not to provide Moslem old people's homes. Moreover, because Bangladeshi people are from a different culture they are frequently denied places on the grounds that the homes are culturally unsuitable: a real 'Catch 22', and yet these people have paid their taxes and are British citizens.

ETHNIC MYTHS

Part of the reason why so little is provided for ethnic minority groups is because of some popular myths. Myths will always exist because they help both the ethnic minority and the host community to come to terms with each other.

The extended family

Like all good myths this one has some basis in reality. The myth is: 'All black and Asian elders live in extended families who provide all the care that is needed.' This is an extremely useful myth because it means no money has to be spent on ethnic minority services, it almost compliments black and Asian people for their devotion to their elders, and it is sustainable because so many black and Asian people seem to live in very large family groupings.

A study from Birmingham showed that a third of West Indian male pensioners lived alone, and that a fifth of Indian pensioners lived alone or in husband/ wife households. The myth is partly true, but a substantial minority of ethnic elders do not live in well-supported large families.

In addition, although the family may wish to support a dependent elder they frequently do not get the sort of support from health and social services that is needed and expected by the white community. For example, it is common to find that incontinence is not managed but ignored by health care professionals. Respite admissions are not arranged, and day care is non-existent.

Learning English

It is tempting to think that communication in the same language would reduce all the problems of service provision. This, too, is a myth. Caribbean elders all speak excellent English, but services that help with their needs have not been forthcoming.

Health and social services are just beginning to realize that they will have to appoint staff with appropriate skills if they are to make any headway. The most appropriate skill in an inner-city area may well be the ability to speak a local minority language.

Assimilation

Linked to the learning-English myth is the **assimilation myth**, which says that in time everything will be all right because the ethnic minorities will become much more like the white community. Interestingly, the Jewish community have retained their cultural identity and have stopped waiting for local services to meet their needs. Jewish homes and hospitals are frequently set up to provide appropriate care.

No demand for the service

This is frequently said by service managers: 'What is the point in trying to provide Halal meals on wheels? There are not enough customers to make it worthwhile.' Provision of Chinese meals on wheels in Tower Hamlets, inner London, only occurred because a Chinese social services manager decided to give it a try. The demand has been huge, even though they cost more than the 'meat and two veg' meals on wheels. Unless an appropriate and sensitive service is provided, demand for it will not emerge.

PROVIDING SENSITIVE SERVICES

The key to a better deal for ethnic elders lies in three directions. The first is in *ethnic monitoring*, which counts the numbers of both service users and providers that come from ethnic minorities. Such information should alert managers to problems with the services they run. It will also help ensure that equal opportunities legislation in employment of black and Asian people is not ignored. The second approach is *positive discrimination* of people from black and Asian groups to fill senior managerial positions. This approach has been highly successful in the USA in producing a better and wider mix of services in multicultural areas. The third approach is to strengthen the existing *self-help and voluntary sector* organizations that work with ethnic elders. This will enable such organizations to take a major role in some aspects of social service provision.

A CHECKLIST FOR ETHNIC ELDERS

It is worth considering the following questions:

1. Are there any interpreters available in your workplace?
2. Does your workplace employ any senior staff from black and Asian backgrounds?
3. Is it possible to get Halal, Chinese, and Kosher meals on wheels in your district?
4. Are signposts, outpatient information, health education material translated in appropriate languages?

5. Are there any ethnic elder patients/clients using your service?

This may be the first step to improving the state of affairs.

Key points

- Many countries have people from a wide range of ethnic groups, all of whom contribute to its social and economic productivity. Ethnic populations are ageing rapidly.
- Services, particularly social, provided for ethnic elders are generally non-existent. This is partly because of a desire, in Britain, for assimilation to occur, and because of an assumption that the extended family will cope with the majority of problems.
- The health problems experienced by ethnic elders (with the exception of tuberculosis) are similar to those of the indigenous population: heart attacks, strokes, diabetes, cataracts.
- Health services would be more sensitive to the needs of ethnic minorities if emphasis were placed on the following: employment of staff from ethnic minorities; use of interpreters; better signposting; provision of health education material in appropriate languages.

FURTHER READING

Ebrahim S, Hillier S. Ethnic minority needs. *Rev Clin Geront* 1991; **1**: 195–199.
Norman A. *Triple Jeopardy: Growing Old in a Second Homeland.* Centre for Policy on Ageing, London, 1985.

32 LEGAL ASPECTS

- Wills
- Refusal to go into hospital
- Mental competence
- Mental Health Act 1983
- National Assistance Act 1948
- The person who can no longer manage

Many elderly people and carers who have lived blameless lives untouched by legal affairs find themselves confronted with legal aspects of old age that can be bewildering. Professionals should be able to provide some guidance.

WILLS

The death of a partner is often a cause for review of finances, and this can be particularly difficult if there is no will. As part of a preventative approach to old age, ensuring that wills have been drawn up is a very practical task. Sometimes it may seem difficult to broach the topic of death with elderly people, but it is often surprising how easily it can be talked about.

REFUSAL TO GO INTO HOSPITAL

Many elderly people have an understandable dread of going into hospital. At best it will be difficult to cope in unfamiliar surroundings; the treatment will be unpleasant; at worst it will end in death or herald the beginning of a terminal phase of severe disability. Confronted with a rational patient who refuses hospital admission, what should be done?

The first step is to discuss the patient's fears. Old workhouse hospitals have almost all disappeared and the patient can be reassured that the care will be up to date. The length of admission can be estimated, and plans made to look after pets, spouses, and the home. The fear of being a burden, of not wanting to cause bother, is often not recognized. The desire to avoid being labelled a 'geriatric' is also strong, and fortunately many departments have changed their names to less derogatory terms such as 'Medicine of Old Age' or 'Health Care of the Elderly'.

The next step, assuming the patient continues in not wishing to go into hospital, is to reassess the purposes of admission. Frequently, the patient's needs are not the prime motive for admission. If nursing care is required, the extent to which family and friends, supported by a district nurse, can manage needs to be considered. The level of staffing on most medical wards is now so low that it is quite feasible to provide as much one-to-one care at home. If the patient requires specific medical treatment, such as an antibiotic, it may be feasible to give it at home. Far too often, family doctors, relatives and other carers place too high a judgement on the ability of hospitals to alter the outcome of disease in elderly people. A home visit by a consultant can often clarify the virtues and risks of hospital admission.

It is important to ensure that the patient is aware of the implications of refusal to admission. It is essential to be clear that refusal of admission is not the same as refusal of treatment, and that the patient can change his mind about admission.

Patients with dementia are a special case when it comes to deciding whether they are competent to decide on management, particularly when this involves hospital admission or institutional care. A demented patient who is presenting major problems in the community (e.g. leaving a gas appliance unlit, wandering, not eating, aggressive behaviour) does not usually wish to be removed from home.

MENTAL COMPETENCE

Social workers and solicitors often ask doctors whether a patient is competent to manage his own affairs, and to make valid decisions for himself. Precise definition of how demented a person has to be before they are considered incompetent is not possible. The best a doctor can do is to make a personal judgement following a full history and examination of the patient, preferably on more than one occasion. The point of history and examination is to ensure that the patient is not suffering from an acute or subacute confusional state, or a depressive illness which may recover, and to assess the severity of any cognitive impairment. A history should be sought of cognitive decline and of behaviour that indicates mental incompetence (for example, over financial matters). The examination must test orientation in time, place and person; short- and long-term memory; insight into problems surrounding the patient; reasoning ability; speech, writing and calculation. In cases where there is any doubt or controversy it may be helpful to ask a clinical psychologist, or another colleague, to carry out a full cognitive assessment and repeat it several months later to demonstrate decline.

MENTAL HEALTH ACT 1983

Often attempts are made using the Mental Health Act to admit a person to an institution against his or her will. This Act was not intended to be used for patients with organic brain disease — dementia is not classed as a treatable mental illness for the purposes of the Act — so strictly should not be used for that purpose. However, in practice there are sections of the Act that can be useful in supporting a commonsense approach to management (see Table 32.1). The Mental Health Act is based on a common law principle; the duty that we all have to help someone who appears to be unable to make an appropriate judgement of their own needs for care.

Table 32.1 Some sections of the Mental Health Act, 1983

Section 2: Admission for assessment or assessment and treatment for up to 28 days. A relative or a social worker together with two doctors (GP plus a psychiatrist usually) must make the recommendation.

Section 3: Admission for treatment for up to 6 months. A relative and social worker must agree that treatment is necessary and the same medical recommendations as in Section2.

Section 4: Emergency admission for up to 72 hours. A relative or social worker together with one doctor (usually GP) must make the recommendation.

Section 5 (2): Allows a patient already receiving treatment in hospital to be kept for up to 72 hours. Recommendation made by the hospital doctor.

Section 5 (4): Allows a patient already receiving treatment in hospital to be kept for up to 6 hours until a doctor can be found. Recommendation usually made by the ward nurse.

Section 136: Allows a police constable to remove a person presumed to have mental illness from a public place to a place of safety for up to 72 hours.

Section 136 is intended to be used by the police if they find someone who they suspect is mentally ill and in need of assessment. It allows for the person to be taken to a suitable place, usually a hospital, for up to 72 hours. Section 4 is also used for emergency admission for 72 hours, but requires a relative or social worker, and a doctor to make the recommendation. It is seldom necessary to use these sections, and since dementia is not classed as a treatable mental illness, it is a questionable practice.

NATIONAL ASSISTANCE ACT 1948

Section 47 of the National Assistance Act is sometimes used to admit elderly people who refuse to go into hospital. The section is specifically for a person who is unable to care for himself, and is not receiving care at home, is suffering with a grave chronic disease (no definition given in the Act) , and is living in insanitary conditions. The Act is not specific about whether the person has to be *both* suffering a grave chronic disease *and* living in insanitory conditions. Different parts of the country vary markedly in their use of this means of admitting elderly people. The safeguards to protect the autonomy of elderly people are weak in this section, and it may be misused to deal with 'difficult' elderly people, rather than those for whom it was intended.

More often the problem is a long-term decline in a demented person's ability to cope, together with behaviour that makes him either neglectful of himself, or unwilling to accept care and attention; this provokes the 'something must be done' phenomenon. It is not usually a good idea to respond to this type of pressure in the middle of the night, since it is likely to be frightening for the patient and the appropriate line of action is usually clearer the next morning. Talk,and reassurance that although the situation has been going on for 'years' you will personally deal with it, are often sufficient.

However, sometimes an alternative used by hard-pressed family doctors is the medical admission of demented patients, with a label of 'toxic confusional state'. While this may solve the family doctor's problem, it is seldom good for the patient. Such patients usually require some form of sheltered accommodation, and inevitably institutional care, unless they have relatives who are willing to look after them. The appropriate action is to contact the duty social worker (phone numbers are available in Accident & Emergency departments and police stations) and request an emergency Part 3 place, provided the person is not acutely sick, or too behaviourally disturbed to be admitted there. In the latter case, admission to a joint psychiatric–medical unit is the best option if available as this allows a full assessment of the patient's mental and physical status. Independent living at home, once lost, is rarely regained, hence the decision to admit to an institution should never be made hastily. Sudden deterioration in

mental or physical state or new features should be considered as possible illness episodes and an expert medical opinion sought — possibly via a domiciliary consultation — before admitting the person to a residential home.

Institutional care is in short supply in many places, and is not the first choice of many demented people. Persuasion to accept institutional care is not easy, and until dementia becomes severe is almost always inappropriate. However, if a relative, or social worker, can take the patient to visit the intended home regularly, say for tea, the transition from home to institutional care can be made much more smoothly. There is a distinct morbidity (translocating effect) associated with rapid and unplanned institutional admissions, especially in the elderly mentally infirm.

THE PERSON WHO CAN NO LONGER MANAGE

The prime consideration is whether a person's affairs are being managed in their interests, or in the interests of someone else. Although the legal mechanisms may seem long-winded, they provide a measure of protection for both the incapable person and the person acting on their behalf.

Court of Protection

The Court of Protection was set up as an office of the Lord Chancellor's department to manage the finances of those who cannot do this for themselves. The majority of people under the Court's protection are elderly people living in institutions. It is usual for a relative, or sometimes a social worker, to apply to the Court for the appointment of a 'receiver'. This is a person nominated to act on behalf of the demented person, and may be a relative.

The procedure for application takes several months to complete, and the expense is relatively high, often running into thousands of pounds, depending on the wealth of the person. If the person has only limited resources, the Court need not always appoint a receiver, but may permit assets to be converted into cash for the care of the person, for example to pay nursing home bills. The advantage of using this system is that it protects relatives, and others, from allegations of not acting in the interests of the demented person. Whenever there is conflict (e.g. between relatives) about the use of a person's money, it is sensible to consider application to the Court of Protection for the appointment of an unbiased receiver.

Power of Attorney

This permits an appointed person to act for another on his or her behalf. The appointee may be able to act in all financial aspects, or may be limited to particular items. It is possible to appoint more than one person as an attorney, which may help ensure that the person's wishes are respected. The document is very straightforward, and only has to be signed and witnessed.

However, a Power of Attorney cannot be used if a person is mentally incapable of understanding its implications. It becomes invalid once a person becomes incapable and so must be replaced by a Court of Protection application.

An Enduring Power of Attorney has now been accepted as a means of permitting an attorney to continue to manage the affairs of a person who has become incompetent. This power of attorney works in the same way, but once the person does become incompetent, the attorney must register enactment of enduring powers with the Court of Protection.

Clearly, enduring powers are open to abuse. If it is thought that an attorney is not acting in the person's interests it is wise to discuss this with the attorney, and if necessary report matters to the Court of Protection. It is relatively common for Power of Attorney to be arranged by a solicitor who has not seen the person (nor assessed their competence), and for arrangements to be made for a relative to manage the person's money. Some relatives are more interested in getting their hands on the money than the care and protection of a dependent person — fortunately there are not too many of them.

Guardianship

Mental Health Act 1983, permits local authority Social Service Departments to provide guardianship to persons suffering from a 'mental disorder' to ensure the welfare of the person, or the protection of others. Guardianships are rarely used for elderly people, and are most widely used for people transferred from long-term hospital care back to the community. Usually the guardian is either a social worker or a relative.

In practice guardians have very little power. They cannot manage a person's affairs, they cannot impose treatment on a person, and they place a duty of ensuring adequate care on the local authority. A further difficulty is the definition of 'mental disorder'. The most common reason for seeking this sort of help for an elderly patient is because of dementia, but some authorities will not recognize dementia as a mental disorder. Not surprisingly they are not much used. However, they are a means of ensuring that vulnerable people's needs for care are met, provided that the person is compliant with advice and support (which is usually the case).

Key points

- Everyone should be encouraged to make a will. Have you made yours?
- When a patient refuses to go into hospital try to allay any fears, reassess the need for hospital admission, consider a home visit by a consultant, and ensure that the patient understands that a change of mind is permissible.
- The Mental Health Act 1983 does not recognize dementia as a 'treatable mental illness' and therefore the Act is not properly used for the compulsory admission of patients with organic brain disease.
- Section 47 of the National Assistance Act 1948 may be used to remove to hospital persons who are unable to care for themselves, are not receiving care at home, are suffering with a grave chronic disease, and are living in insanitary conditions. It offers very little safeguard for the person with none of the review procedures built in to the Mental Health Act 1983.
- The Court of Protection will manage the finances of any elderly person who is no longer able to do this, usually setting up a 'receiver' to act for the person.
- A Power of Attorney can only be instituted if the person has a full understanding of its implications at the time it is made. An Enduring Power of Attorney can be applied for — this is still valid if the person becomes mentally incompetent.
- Guardianships under the Mental Health Act 1983 can be used to ensure the welfare of the person or the protection of others but are rarely used for elderly people.

FURTHER READING

Age Concern. *The Law and Vulnerable Elderly People.* 1986.

Brahams D. Involuntary hospital admission under Section 47 of the National Assistance Act. *Lancet* 1987; **ii**:406.

Briscoe M, Harris B. Compulsory detention in hospital under the Mental Health Act 1983. *Br Med J* 1987; **294**:1141–1144.

33 STROKE

- Diagnosis
- CT scanning
- Acute management
- Rehabilitation
- Long-term follow-up
- Prognosis

A stroke is defined as the sudden onset of a focal or global neurological impairment of over 24 hours duration or, leading to death, of presumed vascular causation. Typically it causes weakness down one side, may cause speech impairment, or may lead to loss of consciousness and rapid death.

DIAGNOSIS

Haemorrhage or thrombosis?

Strokes are caused by two distinct mechanisms. The first is through the blocking or interruption of the blood supply to the brain (thrombosis or embolus); the second is through bursting of blood vessels (haemorrhage). It is possible to subdivide this crude classification further into lacunar stroke (due to blockage of small perforating vessels), cerebral haemorrhage secondary to a bleeding disorder, and stroke secondary to hyperviscosity (e.g. in myeloma or polycythaemia); but the mechanisms remain essentially bleeding or blockage. Over 70 per cent of all strokes are due to thrombosis of arteries, most often the middle cerebral artery. Around 15–20 per cent are due to cerebral haemorrhages, and the remainder are due to rarer causes.

It is impossible to tell which type of stroke has occurred just by looking at the patient because the signs and symptoms are very similar. Management and prognosis of stroke occurring by different mechanisms are also broadly similar.

Errors in diagnosis

When the impairment is weakness down one side of the body there is usually little problem with making the diagnosis: most patients can do it for themselves. However, even here it is possible to be wrong. Table 33.1 shows the common problems that can masquerade as stroke. Errors in diagnosis are common, with up to 15 per cent of admitting doctors wrongly diagnosing a stroke, and an even greater number of primary care doctors getting the diagnosis wrong. Such errors do matter because the treatments for many of the problems that mimic stroke are very different.

Table 33.1 Misdiagnosis of stroke: problems that can confuse

Intercurrent illness with previous stroke
Epileptic fit
Brain tumour: primary or metastases
Brain abscess
Meningitis
Neurosyphilis
Subacute bacterial endocarditis
Subdural haematoma
Hypoglycaemia
Fractured hip/humerus

Occasionally the presentation of stroke is masked. For example, the patient may appear to be suffering with a toxic confusional state with no signs of weakness. The patient may have a speech problem — a dysphasia, without any weakness. These presentations frequently perplex the admitting doctor, and may even lead to an erroneous diagnosis of psychiatric illness. The clue is the sudden onset of the problem with previously normal mental function.

Figure 33.1 A clock face drawing

Subtle signs of brain damage can be helpful in supporting the diagnosis of stroke. One of the best tests to use is the clock drawing. The examiner draws a large circle and asks the patient to put the numbers in to make it appear like a clock face (see Fig. 33.1). The patient is then asked to put the hands in to tell the present time. This is a global task to test cognition, comprehension, vision, hearing, psychomotor skill, writing, use of symbols, and spatial awareness. Inability to perform the task may be due to problems in any of the areas mentioned. Typically this test picks

up patients with parietal lobe damage leading to perceptual impairments — difficulty with spatial awareness, inattention on the hemiplegic side, and hemianopia. (See Fig 33.2)

CT SCANNING

Use of CT scans to make the diagnosis is unnecessary, and in up to a third of cases nothing is found on the CT scan. CT scanning may be helpful if the presentation is atypical or there is real doubt about a tumour, haematoma, or abscess in the brain.

Any patient who has an unusual course to their illness merits consideration for a CT scan. The typical patient who improves over the course of several weeks does not need scanning to confirm the diagnosis.

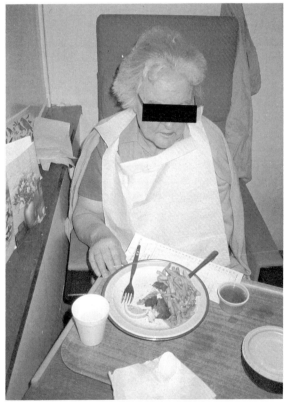

Figure 33.2 This patient shows neglect of the left side of her plate

ACUTE MANAGEMENT

During the acute phase of a stroke a patient is at risk of complications that may hinder recovery or even cause death. The emphasis initially is to protect the airway if the gag reflex has been lost, maintain hydration, avoid pressure sores, regularly turn and position the patient to prevent contractures and orthostatic pneumonia. Patients frequently suffer later because these basic principles are ignored.

There is no medical treatment that will reduce the extent of brain damage or have any beneficial effect on recovery, although the search for new drugs goes on.

REHABILITATION

Stroke recovery occurs over at least three months, and in some cases goes on for over a year. This spontaneous recovery is due to resolution of cerebral oedema surrounding the damaged brain, and relearning of skills. Rehabilitation should start from day one, although often this will be mainly concerned with putting joints through a passive range of movements, giving advice on handling and lifting the patient, and helping with positioning of trunk and limbs both in bed and in a suitable chair.

Swallowing difficulty after stroke may affect up to a third of patients, and it is vital that this is recognized. Often it recovers within two weeks or so, and all that is needed is careful feeding with thickened liquids. In more severe cases it may be necessary to use a nasogastric tube, or even a gastrostomy if the problem persists. Speech therapists are able to give useful advice on management and prognosis as can specialist dentists.

Speech impairment is devastating to most patients, and it is necessary to use whatever modalities of communication that remain. Gestures, noises and communication aids all have a role, and speech therapists are able to advise staff and relatives about how best to communicate and maintain a patient's morale. It is worth remembering that many patients were deaf or had poor sight before the stroke and that correction of these impairments can often aid communication.

Later on, therapy is directed towards achievement of specific goals which tend to recover in a fairly ordered way. The first step is to achieve reasonable sitting balance, and from this the patient moves on to standing and transfers, and then to walking. The usual approach in the UK is based on Bobath methods which encourage bilateral use of the body, rather than the 'natural' tendency for hemiplegic patients to walk in a crab-like unilateral way.

Some patients improve very little, making only a poor recovery. When this occurs it is worth considering whether the patient has made an appropriate recovery in the light of pre-stroke ability and severity of the stroke (see Table 33.2). If the patient seems to have reached a plateau too soon, then it is essential to work out why. This always calls for a thorough reassessment.

Table 33.2 Markers of stroke severity

Unconscious during first 24 hours
Incontinence of urine
Perceptual impairments
Loss of proprioception
Cognitive impairment

The first question to reconsider is the diagnosis. Has the patient really had a stroke, or is the underlying problem a brain tumour? A CT scan may help resolve the diagnosis at this stage. Other questions to ask are: Was the patient fully independent before the stroke (e.g. any evidence of dementia pre-stroke)? Is the patient deaf or blind? Is the patient depressed or dementing secondary to the stroke? Does the patient have unrecognized perceptual difficulties or performance problems (e.g. apraxia of dressing)? Does the patient have an intercurrent illness (e.g. heart failure, urine infection)? All of these are common barriers to rehabilitation and most are treatable.

LONG-TERM FOLLOW-UP

After the acute phase many stroke patients are not followed up and are left to their own management. They are at risk of further strokes, and the main medical priority is to prevent recurrence. The best treatment is to give aspirin (at least 300 mg daily on present evidence) which reduces the chances of a further stroke by about a quarter.

A major task is the prevention of complications of stroke. These are listed in Table 33.3.

Table 33.3 Complications of stroke

Depression
Fractures
Subluxed, painful shoulder
Pressure sores
Contractures
Urinary incontinence/catheter problems
Constipation

Further management should be aimed at maintaining independence and if possible increasing the range of daily activities. Many families try to insulate stroke patients from everyday stress and do far too much for them. This hinders their chances of making a full recovery and encourages them in living a 'sick' role. Any fall in ability should be carefully assessed, and this is usually best done by the day hospital or rehabilitation staff. Any intercurrent illness will make the signs of a stroke much worse, and may fool the doctor into thinking a further stroke has occurred.

PROGNOSIS

It is easy to be misled by the sight of so many hemiplegic patients living out their last years in long-stay hospital wards. The prognosis of stroke is not as bad as it might appear at first (see Fig. 33.3). Death is, of course, possible, and up to half of all people suffering a stroke are dead within six months of onset. Stroke deaths are concentrated within the first few weeks of onset, with primary brain deaths occurring in the first week and subsequent deaths caused largely by complications of stroke (infections, pressure sores, dehydration, heart failure, pulmonary embolus).

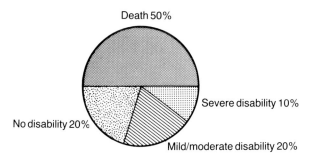

Figure 33.3 Outcome of acute stroke at six months

A difficult problem is deciding how intensively to treat an unconscious stroke patient. Many of them are destined to die because of the severity of their strokes, but it is not possible to predict who with any accuracy. Doctors vary in the extent to which intravenous infusions and antibiotics are given to such patients. In general it is necessary to take both the severity of the stroke, the person's previous ability, and the relatives' view of what should be done into account when making such decisions.

The majority of survivors do get back home and lead reasonable lives, and a minority return to work and a virtually normal life. However, often there are problems of impotence, poor self-image, difficulty concentrating, and the persistent worry of a further stroke that make life much less enjoyable.

Key points

- Strokes are most commonly thrombotic, and the middle cerebral artery is most often affected. Discriminating thromboembolic from haemorrhage stroke is not possible clinically.
- Diagnostic errors are common with up to 15 per cent of patients falsely diagnosed as suffering from a stroke. Among the diseases that mimic stroke are epilepsy (secondary to a previous stroke), space-occupying brain lesions, neurosyphilis, subacute bacterial endocarditis, and hypoglycaemia.
- CT scanning is not essential in every patient with a stroke, but those with an atypical course may be more likely to have non-vascular pathology causing their symptoms and signs.
- No drugs will alter the natural history of an acute stroke. The trend is for patients to either die within the first few weeks of onset, or to make a steady spontaneous recovery.
- Rehabilitation should start from day one and should be goal-directed. Patients who appear to stop progressing early require careful reassessment to detect problems (such as depression, cognitive impairment, hemianopia) that may have been overlooked.
- Long-term follow-up is needed. The aims are: to prevent further strokes by giving aspirin and controlling blood pressure; to prevent complications (depression, contractures, etc.); and to avoid the sick role and over-dependency.
- Recovery is most rapid during the first three months, but can continue for over a year. About a third to one half of all stroke patients die, most within the first six months. About half of all survivors make a reasonable recovery, and only 10 per cent end up in a long-stay hospital ward.

FURTHER READING

Ebrahim S. *Clinical Epidemiology of Stroke.* Oxford University Press, Oxford, 1990.

Wade DT, Hewer RL, Skilbeck CE, David RM. *Stroke: A Critical Approach to Diagnosis, Treatment and Management.* Chapman & Hall, London, 1985.

PART THREE
SERVICES FOR ELDERLY PEOPLE

34 THE MULTIDISCIPLINARY TEAM

- The patient as a team member
- Aspects of teamwork
- Communication
- Key workers
- Team building
- Principles of rehabilitation
- Indicators of success
- The team in primary health care

One of the hallmarks of health care of the elderly is its reliance on teamwork as the main method of working. Working in a team implies that a common purpose is agreed, and that roles, responsibility, accountability and communication are clear.

THE PATIENT AS A TEAM MEMBER

It is essential to remember that the most important member of the team is the patient. This is so easily forgotten when professionals get together, and yet the patient is the focus of the activity. Surely patients should be able to determine their own fate, set their own goals? There can be a tendency for professionals to think they know best. Whenever there is conflict between what the patient wants and what the team decide to do, rehabilitation is highly unlikely to proceed smoothly or successfully.

ASPECTS OF TEAMWORK

Elderly people often have a multiplicity of medical and social problems. Acute illness requiring straightforward drug treatment (e.g. pneumonia) frequently leads to a realization that the patient has other problems that need attention before a safe return home can be arranged. The patient may have difficulty with activities of daily living because of long-standing physical or mental problems. The patient may live in a flat in a block without a lift, and no longer be able to climb the stairs. The patient may be lonely and in need of company.

One response to multiple needs has been for a group of people with different skills to assess the patient in their own ways, and then to share the findings and decide on a plan of action. A *doctor* may help by diagnosing previously unrecognized depression. A *social worker* may help with management by counselling patient and relatives, arranging attendance at a day centre, and home care services such as a home help and meals on wheels. An *occupational therapist* may make assessments of the patient's self-care abilities and institute a programme of practice, together with aids and appliances if necessary. A *physiotherapist* may improve the patient's mobility by improving muscle stength and balance. A *clinical psychologist* may assess the patient's cognitive ability and mood, and set a behavioural management regimen to aid the rehabilitation process. A *nurse* may discover that the patient is incontinent because of poor mobility and depression, and, by counselling and bladder training, help the patient to regain self-respect and continence.

No one discipline possess all the skills that a single elderly patient may require. Teamwork has arisen directly out of the needs of patients.

Teamwork is not always necessary

In some cases, extended teamwork, as described above, may be unnecessary for an elderly patient. A patient with a single-organ disease, and without any other problems, probably does not require the full range of assessments carried out by a multidisciplinary team. Medical and nursing assessments and management are often all that are required. However, amongst the oldest old this is very rarely the case. By the time people reach their high 80s, most have some element of disability, and a team approach is most appropriate.

Who does what and who is in charge?

Effective teamwork is only possible if each member has a clear idea of what their colleagues do (it is to be hoped that team members know what they are meant to do themselves!). See Chapter 42 for an outline of the skills of various health professionals.

In many circumstances some overlap of tasks is both necessary and desirable. Increasingly physiotherapists and occupational therapists share a role of promoting overall independence in activities of daily living rather than focusing on say, mobility and dressing respectively. Nurses in health care of the elderly also have a major role in maintaining practice regimens set up by occupational and physiotherapists. Equally therapists should be prepared to help with nursing management — for example, toileting a patient if it is necessary when they are working with the patient. Doctors and nurses have to be prepared to carry out some of the information-gathering that is considered 'social', because they are in the best position to speak to relatives visiting the patient.

'But that's not my job!'

A team where members start saying this is beginning to fall apart, and probably lacks good leadership. The question of who should lead the team has sometimes been confused with ideas of the leader telling people what to do. This will never work. A good leader knows what team members are capable of, and respects their professional opinions, but should ensure that the team has a clear idea of its goals. The leader must ensure that there is a consensus on tasks, and that any disagreement over who does what is tackled, not avoided.

The doctor as team leader

Many doctors will assert that because of their longer training and high professional status, they should lead the team. Many claim to be trained to be the leader, although in practice this is more likely to mean that they have watched several other consultants be in charge of team meetings.

More important than professional status and number of years at university is the question of continuity and experience. Teams that are run by consultants usually work well because the consultant has a long-term investment in making the team work. Teams run by senior nurses in health care of the elderly work well if the same conditions apply. Teams will never work well if the team leader changes every six months.

COMMUNICATION

In any organization, good communication is essential to efficient and effective working. Teams are no different. The usual method is a regular weekly team meeting. Often this is sufficient, but if patients are changing rapidly more frequent communication is needed. A means of exchange between night and day staff is needed, and between staff who cannot possibly come to every team meeting on every ward — for example, speech therapists, dietitians and clinical psychologists.

Team records

Increasingly, hospital teams are sharing a single,

unified record. Professional boundaries and conflicts have not yet been completely submerged, so all too often the unified record is held along with medical case notes, nursing case notes, occupational therapy and physiotherapy records, and a social work file! A single record, preferably held by the patient and carer, would be the ideal model to follow. Staff would communicate face to face, or by telephone as often as possible, but would also write a note to alert others to what they are thinking.

Case conferences

For patients with complex needs there may be a need to organize a case conference meeting with people from the local community in attendance, with the family and the patient. Such occasions can be very stressful for the patient and family and should not be organized without a very clear purpose. The most common reason for needing a case conference is where there is serious conflict between family and the team about the future prospects for the patient — usually their ability to manage on their own at home after discharge from hospital.

A case conference may reveal previously unknown information that alters the whole perspective of the case. Family members may feel happier when they see that the hospital and community services are working together. They may, however, feel that the professions are closing ranks and conspiring against them. Running a case conference requires a great deal of preparation; it is usually disastrous if the first meeting between consultant and family is at the case conference.

Case conferences should not be used simply to communicate information about a patient's complex needs to community staff. This is a waste of everyone's time. It is usually much wiser to ask district nurses, family doctors and community psychiatric nurses to come in to visit the patient and speak with the ward staff at a time that suits them. Provided everyone is working towards the same goal, with an agreed time scale, this is usually all that is needed in even the most complicated disability.

KEY WORKERS

The idea of a 'key worker' for every patient has grown very popular in some places. Who is a key worker? This person may be a relative or a professional, or sometimes even the patient. Their task is to coordinate the care and treatment that the patient receives, and sometimes to act as an advocate on the patient's behalf.

In practice, the key worker far too often turns out to be the ward sister or charge nurse. This is a reflection of the multiple roles of the nurse, and the amount of contact nurses have with patients. This tends to make the key worker idea less useful in a hospital setting. In the community it may be more useful where a key worker might be a home help, a social worker, a district nurse, a spouse, or a family doctor, depending on the patient's problems.

TEAM BUILDING

Teams are like families if they are working well. They have their ups and downs, but somehow they struggle on. Like a family the team members work best if they get on with each other. The team leader has an important role in ensuring that new team members are accepted, that personality conflicts are not allowed to get out of hand, and that the team develops a measure of self-respect and mastery of its tasks. This may mean substantial time is required for talking through problems. It may be helpful to examine the style of the team from time to time. Persuading other members to 'play' team leader from time to time may be useful in increasing mutual understanding. Changing the means of sharing information — for example, using standardized or computerized records — may increase enthusiasm if the team has hit a low spot.

In general, the best boost for any team is a steady stream of successfully managed patients. Team leaders should ensure that this results in a steady stream of praise.

PRINCIPLES OF REHABILITATION

Setting goals

The purpose of multidisciplinary assessment is to identify problems, and then to define a series of goals that will overcome these problems. For example, a patient with osteoarthritis of the knees may be found to have difficulty climbing stairs, be unable to get into the bath, and have unacceptable side-effects from analgesic medication. The goals may be defined to achieve independent stair-climbing up a full flight, to provide a bathboard, and to provide adequate analgesia by alternative, possibly non-drug, means.

Setting priorities

Whenever there are several interventions to be carried out it is necessary to decide what to do first. The team needs to get together to work out a plan. It might, for example, be best to sort out the analgesia first so that the patient is not in pain, or suffering side-effects. This could permit the physiotherapist to concentrate on improving mobility without pain limiting the progress. Use of a bathboard should probably be deferred because, although the occupational therapist may think it will be needed, it is possible that with increased mobility and better pain relief the patient will not need one.

Monitoring progress

It is essential to decide at the outset what rate of progress will be acceptable. Team members should define in terms of days or weeks how long they think it will take to achieve a goal. If progress appears delayed, this should prompt a reassessment of the patient. Often a previously unidentified problem comes to light — most commonly mild cognitive failure, a small stroke, or depression. Although appropriate goals may have been set, lack of monitoring and failure to reassess are the commonest reasons for rehabilitation failure.

INDICATORS OF SUCCESS

Increasingly rehabilitation teams are required to justify their existence, and some yardstick to measure success or failure is clearly desirable. It is, however, quite difficult to decide what to measure, particularly when patients are so different.

An obvious choice is a patient's ability in activities of daily living (ADL). Successful rehabilitation will lead to patients returning to full ability. However, amongst elderly people this approach is too simplistic. Many have chronic, progressive diseases that will not permit complete restoration of function. Successful rehabilitation may mean some degree of acceptance of disability by the patient, and provision of some

alternative means of achieving the task that cannot be done independently. This may entail a wheelchair for a bilateral amputee, or a good neighbour scheme for a socially isolated housebound person.

The yardstick of success or failure is the extent to which the patient is able to return to a normal lifestyle. Rehabilitation aims to reduce the handicap caused by disease (see Chapter 1 for definitions).

THE TEAM IN PRIMARY HEALTH CARE

Different things have to be said about elderly people in primary health care. The vast majority of a family doctor's patients are well, requiring very little attention from anyone. Furthermore the autonomy of people in their own homes is much more readily respected than in the hospital. Elderly people in their own homes really do know best what it is that they need; they are their own 'key workers'. They may define their needs in general rather than specific terms, and may focus on the family doctor as the route to specific help. A further difference is in time scale. Old people are in hospital for only a short time, and activity is intense. Old people are living in their own homes for most of the time, and the pace of activity need not necessarily be so brisk.

For these reasons, team work in primary health care has evolved in a different way. It is possible for problems to be defined over a period of weeks. The family doctor may see an incontinent patient in his or her surgery, and then ask the continence nurse to call in the following week. The nurse may recommend that as the patient has severe urgency incontinence, a trial of bladder drill be started. The nurse may also ask the community occupational therapist to provide a toilet raise, and a bedside commode. A referral may also be made to the community physiotherapist for help with mobility problems. This sort of teamwork can take place over several months, and does not require regular face-to-face meetings.

When problems start to collect together, and more and more people seem to be involved, that is usually the time to refer the patient from primary care for a specialist opinion. When everything seems to be going wrong, it is vital to get a complete overview. This takes time and is a skilled job, best done by a specialist with the resources of a team, and the training and interest to ensure it is done properly.

<table>
<tr><td>

Key points

- Elderly people benefit from multidisciplinary teamwork because their multiple medical and social problems require the skills of many different professionals. Never forget that the patient is the most important member of the team.
- Effective teamwork requires shared purposes and philosophy, good communication, a willingness to blur professional boundaries, and leadership.
- Rehabilitation comprises the following: multidisciplinary assessment, setting goals and priorities, treatment, and monitoring progress.

</td></tr>
</table>

Success should be measured in terms of the extent to which the patient returns to a normal lifestyle.
- Teamwork in primary health care has evolved in a different way. The time scale is longer, and face-to-face meetings of members of the team less often needed.

FURTHER READING

Andrews K. *Rehabilitation of the Older Adult*. Edward Arnold, London, 1987.

35 COMPREHENSIVE HEALTH CARE

- The role of the generalist
- Organization of health care of the elderly
- Age-related, integrated and needs-related services
- Links with Old Age Psychiatry services
- Misconceptions

The health and social circumstances of elderly people commonly lead to multiple sources of help being required: neurologist, rheumatologist, psychiatrist, social worker, dietitian, and therapists may all be involved in providing aspects of management. Elderly people, as they become frailer, are often required to attend several different places at different times, which can be confusing.

Communication between different specialties, community services, the patient and carers also becomes more complicated the more people are involved. Furthermore, unless a single person is responsible for setting priorities and monitoring progress, conflicts can arise.

As a result of the multiple pathology suffered by elderly people, and the divisions inherent in hospital practice, health services for elderly people aim to provide comprehensive care. This means that each patient is assessed as an individual, a plan of action is decided, and organized by a single team of professionals. Much of the management required is within the competence of the multidisciplinary team, some is not.

THE ROLE OF THE GENERALIST

Health care of the elderly is a specialty for the generalist. Within increasing super-specialization in many medical and surgical specialties, elderly people are at risk of not finding their way to the right professional; or worse, seeing a succession of super-specialists, each of whom gives an opinion on their own bit of the body, leaving the question of who puts all the information together and plans treatment unanswered.

For example, an elderly woman was admitted to a private hospital for a period of bed-rest aimed at reducing her dependent oedema, on the recommendation of her vascular surgeon. On the first night she fell on her way to the lavatory, fracturing her femur. This was repaired by an orthopaedic surgeon and the operation was pronounced a success. However, the patient was not well and her relatives were worried. She slipped into renal failure which prompted a referral to a renal physician who diagnosed dehydration and inappropriate treatment with diuretics, which were stopped. She then suffered with vomiting of altered blood, and a gastroenterologist was called in. He performed an endoscopy, and found multiple small ulcers in her stomach. He recommended treatment with drugs to reduce acid secretion. The patient remained confused, bedfast, and was developing pressure sores. Each specialist had given a thorough assessment of their own organ system, but none had looked at the whole patient. At this stage a geriatrician was called in. The patient had subtle signs of a right hemiparesis, had nominal dysphasia, and was disorientated — she had suffered a stroke. She was transferred to a rehabilitation ward and subsequently made a fair recovery.

Elderly patients need doctors who have had a general and wide training, and enjoy the role of the generalist. However, the main danger of generalists is that they tend to think they can do everything! Knowledge of limitations and the need to refer to specialist colleagues is vital. In the UK very few people in their 70s are referred for renal dialysis, yet renal physicians feel that such patients should not be denied access to life-saving treatment on the basis of age alone. In countries where geriatric medicine has not developed as a major specialty, rates of 'high technology' medical and surgical treatment (e.g. surgery for stroke, use of heart pacemakers and replacement valves, renal dialysis) are much higher than in the UK. Generalists must ensure that access to appropriate (often high-technology) care is not denied to elderly people.

ORGANIZATION OF HEALTH CARE OF THE ELDERLY

Primary health care

Comprehensive health care starts with the primary health care team, which for most elderly people means their family doctor. Many elderly people have the good fortune to be looked after by a doctor who has known them for many years, and has an understanding of how the individual has responded to illness in the past. The family doctor also knows much of the background relationships in the family, about the health of a spouse, and about the local services and environment.

Family doctors are not the only primary health care resource. It is possible to arrange community nursing support in the patient's home. Nursing equipment, including mattresses to combat pressure sores, can be provided at short notice. Community physiotherapists can be asked to assess and treat the patient at home. Social services can be asked to arrange home care services, and a community occupational therapist can provide aids, appliances and home modifications. However, all of this takes time to organize and some family doctors do not do it well.

The most important element in primary health care is appropriate training in health care of the elderly for family doctors and community nurses. Most family doctors now accept that special training in child health is essential for competent treatment of babies and children, and training in obstetrics is legally required before family doctors are allowed to manage pregnancy. Similarly, trainees in primary health care, community nurses, and health visitors are increasingly gaining experience in health care of the elderly.

Primary care and hospital

Another essential for comprehensive health care is a good working relationship with local hospital services for elderly people. The interface between community and hospital is always a source of potential communication and responsibility problems. Easy access to the hospital departments is essential — this means high-quality secretarial staff who understand the constraints on family doctors, liberal use of phone answering machines, mobile phones, faxes and accessible consultant and junior staff using 'bleeps' when they are on duty. Equally, modern primary health care has to invest in good communication systems. Economizing by manning telephones for only three or four hours a day, and heavy use of deputizing services, is not compatible with good communications.

Increasingly, geriatricians are experimenting with styles of practice that take them into closer contact with primary health care teams. Using a model borrowed from psychiatric practice, some geriatricians are carrying out clinics in health centres. Many geriatricians have links with local authority old people's homes, giving an informal service to the home and advice to family doctors about residents. Other possibilities are for geriatricians to conduct 'problem case' discussion groups with primary health care teams regularly, or to appoint liaison nursing staff to hospital teams who visit patients known to the hospital service, as well as visiting the patients' family doctors and nurses.

AGE-RELATED, INTEGRATED AND NEEDS-RELATED SERVICES

The relationship between geriatric medicine and general (internal) medicine has to be clear within a hospital. When elderly patients are admitted it is necessary to decide which service should look after them. In the past, geriatric medical services operated in isolation, taking those patients referred to them as the supply of beds determined. This frequently led to long waiting lists, and a feeling among both primary health care and the rest of the hospital that geriatric medicine was not working efficiently.

To combat this style of practice several different models of care have arisen. One of the earliest attempts to rationalize the services was the use of *an age cut-off*, usually set at 75 years: everyone over 75 is referred to the geriatric medical service and those under 75 are referred to the general medical service. Obviously, some patients under 75 have multiple pathology and need the teamwork approach adopted by geriatric medicine. By contrast, some people over 75 are 'biologically' young with single problems that might be equally well, or better, managed by general medicine. Age-related services always run the risk that they will offer a second-rate service to elderly people, managing them in worse wards, with fewer medical and nursing staff. In addition, hospitals using this model are committed to having a double complement of staff on call — geriatric and general medical.

An alternative model is that based on *integration*. Here geriatricians are part of the general medical service. In the same way that most general physicians have a sub-specialty interest, the geriatrician is considered to be a general physician with an interest in the elderly. This model ensures that geriatricians have full access to high-technology medicine, and more importantly use similar wards and junior medical and nursing staff as other physicians. A two-tier service cannot occur.

Another model is based on the *needs-related* approach. Geriatricians take those patients who most need their style of practice, and elderly patients who have single problems are managed by the general medical service. This type of arrangement can end up

providing a service only to the most difficult patients, which puts extra pressure on nursing and therapy staff. Its image may become that of a 'takeaway service', with the geriatrician simply viewed as a convenient disposal route for difficult patients.

However, this approach ensures that the scarce skills of the geriatrician are not diluted by time spent managing the relatively easy problems of acute internal medicine.

In practice, the type of relationship with general medicine will be dictated by local circumstances and the interests and training of geriatricians. In smaller district general hospitals it makes good sense to adopt an integrated pattern of care, sharing resources between the small number of physicians and geriatricians. In large hospitals an age-related model may be more feasible provided adequate medical and nursing staff can be allocated to the geriatric service, and physicians are willing to forgo much of the general medical acute work.

The needs-related service is often in place where relationships between geriatric and general medicine have been poor in the past. To ensure that those acutely ill elderly patients who need to be managed by a geriatrician are dealt with appropriately, some form of limited integration can be organized. This usually involves the pairing of general medicine teams with a geriatrician. The geriatrician then provides the care for some or all of the elderly patients admitted acutely, using the general medical wards and staff. In most circumstances, the needs-related model is the best option for patients.

LINKS WITH OLD AGE PSYCHIATRY SERVICES

Old Age Psychiatry has blossomed as a separate sub-specialty in psychiatry over the last two decades. This can be seen as a deliberate response, similar to geriatric medicine, to provide services for a growing patient group with specific problems requiring a different style of management.

An ideal model of collaboration is for combined departments of geriatrics and old age psychiatry — departments of health care of the elderly. Primary health care, hospital colleagues, and other agencies are never in any doubt about where to refer. A single department acts as the entry point into the service. Thereafter care may be supervised by whichever specialist is most appropriate, or if necessary, by both.

However, this model is the exception rather than the rule. Old age psychiatrists have a foot in both the psychiatry and geriatric medical camps, but most of them have preferred to stay within psychiatry. This is unfortunate because much of the psychiatric 'action' among elderly people is in the district general hospital. The presentation of illness in old people often has a psychiatric flavour, leading to some doubt about where the patient should be referred. With dementia syndromes, help is often sought from a geriatrician or physician because of a concurrent physical illness, yet the management of the dementia syndrome is often of higher priority and importance than the physical illness, and requires the skills and resources of old age psychiatry.

Collaboration need not involve fully integrated services. It may be simply informal and episodic as the need arises, or may be done by holding joint ward rounds regularly. It is essential that there is a relationship of some sort between geriatric medicine and old age psychiatry to avoid the buck passing that can occur with patients suffering a mixture of physical and psychiatric problems.

Old age psychiatry is a very young specialty which is developing rapidly. Already the emphasis in training is for old age psychiatrists to have some senior level geriatric medical experience. Equally all geriatricians should have some training in psychiatry. These developments should bring the two specialties closer together, and, with increased resource limitations, should encourage sharing of facilities like day hospitals, outpatient clinics, secretarial and other staff. Greater collaboration can only benefit patients.

MISCONCEPTIONS

There is still much confusion in the minds of both professional staff and the general public about the role of health care of the elderly. The most popular misconception is that the service exists only for the provision of long-stay beds for the very frail. In the past, geriatricians did indeed have control of very large numbers of long-stay beds, often in hospitals several miles from the main district hospital. Many of these hospitals have now shut, and the pool of long-stay beds is shrinking year by year. Modern health care of the elderly aims to provide a wide range of services for elderly people (see Table 35.1).

The range of tasks is daunting and not all are done with equal competence or enthusiasm. Preventive

health care is seldom part of the service on offer, and increasingly it is recognized that prevention in old age is of value. The relationship with the private sector is not well developed in most parts of the UK. This large sector of care for very frail people is largely ignored by most departments of health care of the elderly. The

Table 35.1 Services provided by a department for health care of the elderly

Hospital inpatients
Acute treatment
Rehabilitation
Shared management with Old Age Psychiatry
Shared management with Orthopaedics
Shared management with General Medicine
Long-stay hospital patients
Hospital outpatients
General clinics
Shared clinics: diabetes, Parkinson's disease
Memory clinic
Continence clinic
Day Hospital
Medical/rehabilitation
Psychiatric
Liaison with community services
Home visits
Liaison nursing
Part 3 home visits
Clinics in general practice
Training
Trainees in general practice/general medicine
Nursing
Care staff in Part 3 homes
Social work trainees

challenge of the increasing number of very frail elderly people managed in the community has also yet to be faced by most departments. It is unrealistic to imagine that shifting the place of care of patients from hospital long-stay to the private sector or into patients' own homes will alter their need for the attentions of specialists in health care of the elderly.

Key points

- Elderly patients require a generalist to ensure that multiple pathology does not lead to multiple referrals, opinions, and dilution of responsibility.
- The primary health care team provides a comprehensive approach, but many general practitioners require more training in health care of the elderly.
- Liaison between primary and hospital services is vital, with easy communication and clear lines of referral.
- Sharing of work between general (internal) and geriatric medicine has evolved in three main ways:

age-related (e.g. 75+ cut off); integrated (i.e. no separate admission system); and needs-related (GP decides where to refer). There is no 'best' way of sharing the work; each method has advantages and disadvantages.

- Links with Old Age Psychiatry services are crucial for patients with a mixed medical/psychiatric presentation.
- Health Care of the Elderly services are wide ranging and aim to be innovative and comprehensive to meet the challenges of an increasingly frail and dependent population.

FURTHER READING

Arie T (ed.). *Health Care of the Elderly*. Croom Helm, London, 1980.

36 THE DAY HOSPITAL

- Medical day hospitals
- Psychiatric day hospitals
- The multidisciplinary team
- Problems and the future

Borrowing the concept from Russia, UK psychiatrists developed day hospitals as places where treatment and management could continue while the patient lived at home. This successful idea spread to the care of the elderly at the inception of the NHS and now day hospitals form part of the spectrum of care options for most departments of health care of the elderly. The term *day hospital* is often confused with *day centre* (a Social Service resource providing meals, diversional therapy and companionship). A day hospital is an NHS unit which is usually part of a Health Care of the Elderly department and either a medical or psychiatric facility. A few day hospitals intentionally mix their clientele; hence the range of expertise of their staff. Day hospitals should be on the district general hospital site.

MEDICAL DAY HOSPITALS

Traditionally the aim is to provide an assessment unit where medical and rehabilitation treatments can be performed whilst keeping the patient living in the community (at home or in Part 3 accommodation). This is achieved by providing the following:

1. concentration on rehabilitation but especially the maintenance of skills needed in daily living;
2. medical plus multidisciplinary team assessment, investigations and team follow-up of the 'problem list';
3. regular (short-term) review of problems, monitoring of medical, therapy and social needs;
4. advice based on knowledge base of 'networks' and often involving home visits and liaison with community teams.
5. supporting the carer.

Referrals tend to reflect the rehabilitative nature of most day hospitals, and mobility problems form a large subsection of attenders (see Table 36.1). Problems such as urinary incontinence, weight loss, or inability to cope, often account for another group. One-problem cases, by virtue of the multidisciplinary nature of the set-up, are in the minority; yet when more time is needed than can be given in the outpatients clinic, the day hospital can be invaluable (e.g. for intermittent blood transfusions, and one-off procedures). Patients who have 'failed' on discharge previously often form another group of attenders.

Table 36.1 Problems that can be well managed at a day hospital

Assessment of falls
Mobility (stroke, Parkinson's disease, arthritis)
Assessment of weight loss/incontinence/constipation
'Inability to cope' syndrome
Difficult discharges/carer, client anxiety
Procedures (intermittent blood transfusion, etc.)
Chronic confusion/'dementia' screen
Problems with activities of daily living (transfers, toileting, cooking, etc.)
Clients with multiple problems (e.g. ulcers, drug compliance, COAD)

PSYCHIATRIC DAY HOSPITALS

The 'provision' list is basically the same as for medical day hospitals, with the added emphasis on the mental state of the patient. Some psychiatric day hospitals incorporate *memory clinics* in the range of assessment features offered. Memory clinics investigate people presenting with the symptom of memory impairment and thus help in the early detection of possible causes including dementia. Some clinics accept self-referrals, but most are via health care workers, especially GPs. The standard core of professional expertise within a memory clinic consists of a clinical psychologist, physician and psychiatrist. These people usually assess the referral independently and collate their data to a cumulative profile (nursing input is helpful and social work involvement extremely valuable). The psychologist assesses any memory loss via testing instruments (e.g. the Kendrick battery) and now computer-assisted tests. The physician excludes treatable causes of memory loss (e.g. hypothroidism) and the psychiatrist assesses mental state (e.g. affective disorders).

Some psychiatric day hospitals further subdivide into those that deal with affective disorders such as depression and those that deal with mainly organic problems (e.g. dementia). As a generalization, people attending psychiatric day hospitals tend to be mobile and the team is geared to the more physically fit and ambulant person. Medical day hospital patients tend to be more frail and are often immobile. The two populations overlap however causing conflict when rigid definitions concerning attendance criteria have to be adhered to.

'Social' care is rarely a stated aim within day hospital attendance criteria yet most day hospitals have a small group of long-term attenders who cannot be discharged and who are too frail or difficult for a day centre. This social care role relieves carers and may keep the person temporarily or permanently out of an institution. Long-term attenders have cost implications, and if a day hospital accumulates many such patients the multidisciplinary team can lose morale and be unable to accept new referrals owing to lack of space.

THE MULTIDISCIPLINARY TEAM

Just as the multidisciplinary team is essential to effective management and discharge in a ward setting the same is true in the day hospital. Most day hospitals have a manager or organizer, often a nurse or occupational therapist by training. The range of 'core' expertise in most medical day hospitals includes medical (usually junior), nursing, occupational therapy, social work and physiotherapy. A standard routine (dependent on the referral problem) involves a 'medical' clerking with nursing, OT and mobility assessment. There are usually weekly meetings to review and agree the 'problem' list and to consider referral to other agencies serving a day hospital (dietitian, speech therapy, chiropody, dentist, continence adviser, etc.). Attendance rates are decided and treatment plans organized, with weekly meetings to assess progress until discharge can be contemplated.

PROBLEMS AND THE FUTURE

Recently, however, day hospitals have come under more critical scrutiny, not only with regard to their role but also to their cost-effectiveness. In many areas their role has become rigid and they have not developed as the client/patient needs have altered. There has been a downward shift in dependency with increasingly frailer people living at home or in Part 3 accommodation (displacing the less frail type of client found there 10 years ago). Most day hospital attenders need transport, which has proved difficult. Patients often arrive late, leave early, and spend many hours 'touring' their local district. Dedicated ambulances with escorts are an essential element to a successful day hospital.

The role of carers may not be fully appreciated and their needs not assessed. Day hospitals should develop carer support groups and possibly run a 'rolling' series of talks aimed at carers and other non-professional groups to help them understand ageing, disability and the common diseases. Day hospitals need to 'communicate' more effectively. This can be directed towards the patient and carer via explanatory booklets and a 'diary' — a communication notebook kept by the patient, in which day hospital staff note treatments performed and changes in medication, and into which the patient and carer write when the need arises at home. All day hospital staff need to assess and monitor their effective contact with patients, surveys indicating communication between staff and patients to be poor and they also reveal a lamentable lack of actual contact time with patients in all disciplines.

Day hospitals will not survive the economic strait-jacket unless they can demonstrate a cost-effective niche in the delivery of health care. This means that every day hospital has to evaluate its method of working, its acceptance criteria, the costs of treatment and transport, throughput of patients, etc. Day hospitals must adapt to changing circumstances, perhaps acting as education and resource centres (the base for continence advisers, chiropody, dental and memory clinics), and rapid assessment for community care and general practice patients. Close cooperation with psychiatry and other specialties may enable premises to be used more effectively. For example, there could be combined days for the elderly mentally ill (EMI), plus EMI with medical problems, joint clinics with neurology (Parkinson's disease and stroke) and orthopoedics. Increasingly the NHS will move away from the day-care/out-patient model. The US concept of 'polyclinics' (numerous specialties cooperating and allowing multiple assessments quickly and efficiently in one geographical area) is gaining support. The concept of day hospitals being open in the evening/weekends with varied use will develop. Liaison with Social Services is another area for study: there are already joint premises with day hospital, day centre and luncheon club under the same roof but often organized and run separately.

Day hospitals for the elderly are a unique and important facet in health care. Although economic factors will play their part, sufficient attention will have to be paid to the patient and client requirements and satisfaction levels compared with the alternatives. Hospital-at-home schemes are not always appropriate and need closer economic appraisal. Care in hospital is expensive and not 'user friendly'; most people want to be at home. Day hospitals can bridge the gap between what is acceptable to the patient (staying at home or getting home sooner) yet fulfilling the professional needs of treatment and maintenance programmes. Transport, client mix, function, opening hours and staff levels and mix are all comparatively flexible parameters allowing day hospitals to adapt and flourish.

Key points

- A day hospital is an NHS resource (day centres are run by Social Services).
- Day hospitals provide multidisciplinary assessment.
- There is a concentration on rehabilitation and the skills needed in daily living.
- Psychiatric day hospitals may be organic (dementia), functional (depression) or both and may incorporate a memory clinic.
- Long-term attenders are a reality but every endeavour should be made to keep the numbers low.
- Dedicated ambulances are an essential element to successful working.
- Carer groups are an important aspect.

FURTHER READING

Brocklehurst JC, Tucker JS *Progress in Geriatric Day Care*. King Edwards Hospital Fund for London, 1980.

Maczka K. *Occupational Therapists' Reference Book of the Bethnal Green Day Hospital*. British Association of Occupational Therapists, 1988.

37 SEVERE CHRONIC DISABILITY

- Services for the disabled
- A typical day
- The carers: formal and informal
- Respite care or recurring admission?
- Who needs a long-stay hospital or nursing home?
- Making the best of institutional care

Medicine seems to teach us that *cure* is the only outcome worth considering. Patients who are not cured are failures, and highlight the doctor's impotence to solve their problems. This is simplistic, but does explain some of the attitudes surrounding patients with severe chronic diseases. In some way, they are not 'proper' patients because they do not get better; their problems are redefined as 'social' to ensure that doctors do not have to get involved. Often such patients are passed on to geriatric services because they can 'no longer be helped'.

Even in a rehabilitation unit, patients who do not do well are considered to be 'failures'. They fail to conform to the expectations of professionals and can suffer because of this. Less interest is taken in their futures, and little thought given to how they, and those around them, will cope.

SERVICES FOR THE DISABLED

Organizing services requires careful assessment. The first step is almost always a team assessment of disease processes, functional ability, continence, cognition and personality, mobility, and social background. Once a complete picture of the relative strengths and weaknesses of the person has been put together it is essential to decide *with the person and family* what will be needed.

Sometimes medical treatment will continue to be needed for deteriorating chronic diseases such as heart failure, arthritis, or Parkinson's disease. Usually rehabilitation will be needed, either to achieve a specific goal, or to maintain a level of ability. Social work is vital, but often a very limited resource. The counselling tasks are as important as providing information on welfare benefits and home care services but are time consuming. Access to all these services is extremely limited in institutions, particularly in the private sector, and almost as poor for people living at home.

A TYPICAL DAY

The best approach to thinking and acting for people with disability is to consider their typical day — the full 24 hours. Start with getting up in the morning, and try to relate what you would do with what the person might want to do, and can do. For each disability it is necessary to think of some way around the disability, thus creating ability. This is usually

tion now has showrooms where equipment can be seen and tested, and local authority occupational therapy departments are setting up Aids and Appliances Centres. These may facilitate choice and loans of equipment until the person knows whether

Table 37.1 The disabled person's morning

	Task	Substitutes
Waking up	Orientation: time Alert others Hot drink	Alarm clock radio Radio on 'Teasmade'/thermos, may need straw
Getting out of bed	Assisted transfer to wheelchair	Done by husband + mobile hoist May need nurse if spouse unwell or unable
Going to lavatory	Assisted transfer to lavatory	Done by spouse/toilet raise + rails, one-handed paper dispenser, one-handed suppository applicator
Shower	All-over wash	Modified shower room, with seat, soap on a rope, Towel dressing gown + help from spouse
Breakfast	Making breakfast	Assist spouse using modified breadboard, electric toaster, and tea dispenser
	Eating	Able to manage independently
Daily news	Read newspaper, switch radio/ TV channels	Spouse reads items out loud Use hand held channel changer
Arrival of friends	Open front door, open curtains, move to living room	Remote control door lock + video camera Environmental control electronics: power points, appliances Self-propelled wheelchair

done by getting a relative or friend to stand in for the person. However, with more thought and creativity, and advances in technology, disabled people can be given more autonomy, and their dependence on other people reduced — if that is what they and those around them want (see Table 37.1).

The key to producing a viable plan for disabled people is to involve them and their relatives in deciding what is wanted. For example, some people may simply want to spend the whole morning in bed, only getting out to go to the lavatory. They may wish to conserve their energy for later in the day, or may simply see little point in being up for no obvious reason, however much it accords with a professional view of how the morning should be spent. Some people may prefer to be incontinent of faeces, using an incontinence pad, rather than go through the business of two transfers, a cold lavatory, and an undignified wipe of the bottom by a close relative. The secret is to ask the person, and not impose artifical standards.

Equipment and adaptations

A major difficulty in deciding what would be useful is the limited opportunity for 'road-testing' expensive pieces of equipment. The Disabled Living Founda-

the item really suits.

Given the individual nature of disability and handicap it is very difficult to give a formula plan of action that will suit every patient. There are so many different aids and appliances that may help. Keeping up to date with changes is the task of occupational therapists, and their help should always be sought when considering equipment.

Lifting

These tasks are frequently too much for a frail carer. In some cases, a small hoist at home will make the difference between success and failure of home care. The range of hoists is large, and style of slings, their size and manoeuvrability also vary. Sometimes a hoist is not the answer, but advice about lifting, a transfer board, a higher chair may be all that is needed.

Mobility aids

Assessment by a physiotherapist and occupational therapist working together is the best means of ensuring the patient gets a good deal out of mobility aids.

Wheelchairs are often provided but not used as they are not a complete solution to the problem of immobility. The first decision is about who will be providing the effort — patient or carer. If the chair is exclusively for outings with the rest of the family, a collapsible assisted wheelchair is best. If the patient is going to propel herself, then who will assist with transfer into the chair, will it fit through doorways, and does the patient have sufficient reserves of stamina?

Inspection of wheelchairs should be systematic: brakes, tyre inflation, foot plates and seat padding should all be examined. Walking frames are robust and need little maintenance, but handles do crack and the collapsing type may prove unstable for some patients. Walking sticks can transform a patient with osteoarthrosis of the hip, and boost confidence. The length is important. It is best measured by inverting the stick and placing it alongside the patient's wrist: the correct length should correspond to the crease of the wrist joint. Quad sticks (those with four legs at the base) used to be popular for patients who had suffered strokes but tend to encourage a poor walking pattern and are now not often used.

THE CARERS: FORMAL AND INFORMAL

A major part of the care plan for people with complex severe disability is attention to the needs of the carers. Carers include all of those people, both professional and family, who help the disabled person. Professional carers gain support and confidence in the tasks they do through their training and experience. They often work in groups which provide extra psychological and practical support when work gets tough.

For informal carers — wives, husbands, children, friends and neighbours — the set-up is very different. There is little recognized training for caring, no support and no extra help when things get difficult. Many carers are elderly themselves and have their own health problems and yet they are often expected to do a job of work that few health professionals would consider feasible. Recently national and local carer networks have been set up to increase the attention given to the problems of carers, and increase the

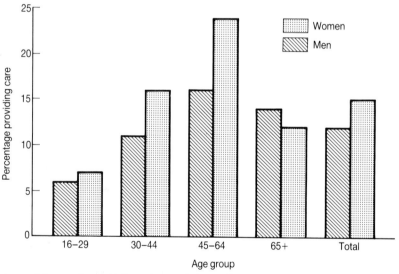

Figure 37.1 Breakdown of the numbers of informal carers in Britain by age group; 1.4 million carers spend at least 20 hours a week caring (General Household Survey, 1985)

Battery-operated wheelchairs and tricycles are expensive and often bought with little practical assessment. This is a pity since they are of only limited use and careful assessment will demonstrate who will benefit. Stair lifts, too, are expensive to fit and may turn out to be inappropriate for many patients.

number of support and training schemes available.

It is vital to recognize the essential resource of informal carers. Without them the health and social services would collapse, but as a society we place so little value on their role that we do not pay them and give scant attention to their views.

In general, carers need training to carry out the tasks of assisting disabled people. The best training is one-to-one with a therapist and carried out in the home. This gives the carer the confidence to ask about practical problems: how do I get him onto the toilet here? how do I get him into this bed? The ideal situation of the hospital is so far removed from most people's homes that it only gives a limited view of what the person will be able to do at home.

RESPITE CARE OR RECURRING ADMISSION?

Carers need a break from caring, and disabled people may need breaks from their carers, particularly for periods of 'top-up' rehabilitation and nursing care. Flexible respite is frequently asked for but unfortunately is often not available. Respite for the carer may be given by admission of the disabled person to hospital or a Part 3 old people's home (depending on the physical and mental condition of the person) for a week or two, by a regular cycle of admissions (e.g. two weeks in and six weeks out), or by occasional nights spent as an in-patient, or by a night or day-time sitter who will cover for the carer.

The nature of respite care needs better definition. In some cases it is simply to give carers a break from the burden of caring. However, it is often better to think of it as a recurring admission to a rehabilitation environment where the patient may benefit from team assessment and a short course of treatment aimed at maintenance of function. This can be a more acceptable reason for admission for many carers who may find it difficult to accept their own needs for support and respite.

WHO NEEDS A LONG-STAY HOSPITAL OR NURSING HOME?

The answer varies according to where you live. In some parts of the world (e.g. the UK, New Zealand) where there are financial incentives to use private and public sector care for disabled elderly people, large numbers find themselves in institutions. In general most disabled people want to live in their own homes and lead as normal a life as possible. The aim therefore should be to promote care within the person's home.

Table 37.2 Reasons for living in an institution

Inadequate pre-admission assessment
Lack of a carer
Unsuitable housing
Behaviour (e.g. faecal smearing or screaming)
Severe disability
Poor community services
Wishes of the person
Financial incentives (state subsidies)

Even amongst the most severely disabled elderly, a fair proportion (30 per cent) can be looked after at home. The reasons why many are in institutions are shown in Table 37.2.

Among those unfortunate people with moderate to severe dementia syndromes it is worth noting that for a proportion no amount of 'care in the community' can avoid the need for institutional care. Such people often need total supervision to avoid catastrophes or neglect. At present we tolerate a large degree of neglect and deal with crises as they arise, which does not constitute good quality care.

As the level of disability increases, care needs also increase. It is likely that at some point it becomes cheaper to look after a person in an institution rather than at home. This point is usually reached when the person needs help more often than every 4–6 hours, or requires help during the night, and has no immediate informal, *free* carer. Increasingly the needs of younger chronically disabled are being met by setting up group living homes, with resident care staff. For the elderly we are a long way from offering this sort of choice.

MAKING THE BEST OF INSTITUTIONAL CARE

It is possible to make an institution more homely, and this is best done by removing many of those aspects of hospitals and nursing homes that are designed to suit staff and 'the system'. The first question to ask concerns aspects of the care given to patients is: 'In whose interests is this done?' For example, in bathing routines: Is the preference for a bath or shower taken into account? Does the frequency of bathing match the person's usual practice? Is privacy possible? The same questions should be asked of all aspects of the resident's day. If there is any doubt, it usually means that patterns of care are done to suit staff rather than residents. One of the best examples of what can be done with long stay wards is provided by the

Bolingbroke Hospital in South West London, which owes much to the enthusiasm of Professor Peter Millard.

Individualism

A further approach is to try to imagine what it would be like to live in the institution yourself. What things would irritate you? What could you live with? What would you change? Perhaps the most important aspect of care is the extent to which individualism is accepted and encouraged. Respect for individuals does not just happen, it has to be worked at. Simply seeing a frail, white-haired woman as an individual can be difficult. She looks just the same as the other 20 women on the ward. The key is to focus on the person's life history, to know what they looked like in their prime, to ensure that the person's own clothes are used, that momentos and photos are on display.

Autonomy

Autonomy is also vital. It is easy to confuse the two concepts of autonomy and dependency, assuming that dependent people are incapable of exerting autonomy (or choice) over events. Dependency is a relationship between a person, another person(s), and an environment. Obviously many people without disability are dependent to some extent on others. The dependency relationship should not lead to removal of choice. In hospitals, it has become more and more difficult to encourage autonomy amongst the ever frailer residents, most of whom have some degree of cognitive impairment. It is easier in old people's homes and in sheltered accommodation as people are in greater day-to-day control of their lives and are usually less intellectually impaired.

Routines

Fixed routines are the hallmark of institutional practice and should be avoided where they contribute nothing to residents' well-being. Waking-up times and bed-times should be decided by individual preference and not routine, whereas mealtimes give shape to the day, should be pleasurable, and are an opportunity for social engagement. Some variation in the residents' day is valuable, giving the idea of something to look forward to, something to enjoy and live for.

A ward in a hospital may be 28 beds, and a home may have 50 residents. This does not mean that every activity in the institution has to be done in these large groups. Smaller groupings can be more informal and more spontaneous, and certainly allow care staff to get to know residents better.

Privacy

Privacy in an institution can be a rare commodity. Nothing is private, not even a bath or bowel action. It is worth considering how privacy can be maintained. More single rooms, fewer shared bathrooms and lavatories would all help. Greater use of personal stereos and televisons might help reduce the noise pollution in many institutions, which can be difficult for some residents to endure. Perhaps an overprotective attitude on the part of staff leads to a desire to reduce risk of falling, or of dying, without someone knowing and seeing. In practice the use of name plates and bells on residents' doors, staff who encourage residents to exert their choices and preferences, and acceptance of a degree of risk go some way to improving privacy.

Relatives and friends

Involvement of relatives and friends is essential to running a happy institution. Relatives are anxious to ensure that standards are high, but may be viewed as trouble-makers by busy, pressured staff. Relatives are a major resource in an institution, and are often the residents' only link with the outside world. Their comments should be taken seriously, complaints acted upon. Their involvement in the day-to-day care of residents should be encouraged. It is important that relatives get to do some of the nice things and the nasty things; taking granny out for a drink in the garden is enjoyable for everyone, but taking her to the lavatory, or cutting her finger nails, should not be viewed as a strictly nursing task. Relatives should be encouraged to view the institution as a home from home, where they can make choices themselves, and have a degree of control over what happens.

Key points

- Chronically disabled people require a diary for their day, establishing what has to be done and by whom.
- People should be allowed to 'road test' expensive equipment (such as hoists, battery wheelchairs) prior to deciding whether to make an order.

- Carers require much greater consideration for all the free care provided. Their needs are for training and for respite from caring.
- Long-term institutional care is often used by people who do not require it. Reasons include financial incentives through state subsidies, inadequate pre-admission assessment, and lack of a carer.
- Avoiding the worst aspects of institutional care requires the question 'in whose interests is this done?' to be asked of all practices (e.g. mealtimes, bathing regimens, bedroom allocation).
- Autonomy should not be confused with dependency. Dependent people should be able to exert their own autonomy (choice). Needs for privacy do not disappear in institutions.
- Relatives and friends should be actively engaged in the running of the institution.

FURTHER READING

Denham M (ed.). *Care of the Long-Stay Elderly Patient*, 2nd edn. Chapman & Hall, London, 1990.

Mulley G. *Everyday Aids and Appliances*. British Medical Journal, London, 1989.

38 PREVENTION IN OLD AGE

- Primary prevention
- The new GP contract
- Screening
- Case finding and surveillance
- Tertiary prevention

'Prevention is better than cure' is a well established dogma. For elderly people, the opportunities for prevention may seem limited compared with those for children and younger adults. However, survival has increased so much in the last century that the majority of people who reach retirement can expect to live another 15 to 20 years. This is a long time, and the prevention of diseases during this time is becoming much more relevant. Also, the increased levels of disease and disability amongst the very old suggest that ways of preventing problems must be looked for and implemented.

Table 38.1 summarizes the three-pronged approach discussed in this chapter.

Table 38.1 Classification of prevention

Primary
Prevention of disease occurrence (e.g. immunization)

Secondary
Early detection of disease (e.g. screening for cancers)

Tertiary
Prevention of complications of established disease (e.g. contractures after stroke)

PRIMARY PREVENTION

There are many diseases that are either common among elderly people, or can be easily prevented. The modern health promotion movement has emphasized the things that people can do for themselves to prevent ill-health, by means of lifestyle modification. Elderly people are as keen as younger adults to achieve greater control over their destiny, and wish to be involved in anti-smoking, exercise and dietary changes. Unfortunately many health professionals are rather negative in their attitudes, which leads to health promotion for elderly people being seen as a low priority.

Immunization

We tend to think of infectious diseases as affecting only babies and children and are used to ensuring that they get their 'jabs'. However, rare diseases like tetanus now occur to any extent only amongst elderly people; and others, such as influenza and pneumococcal pneumonia, cause serious levels of mortality only among the elderly. Therefore there are good reasons to ensure that elderly people get their jabs as well.

Exercise

The panacea for all the ills of old age is now exercise. The evidence that exercise is of benefit to elderly people is incomplete, and would not satisfy every scientist. Doubts remain over how much exercise to recommend, what type of exercise, what risks might be involved and the precise benefits that might be expected. Well-designed experimental trials will be needed to give answers to these questions.

However, the health professional has to decide what to do now, not when all the evidence has been collected and sifted. There are beneficial effects on well-being and physical fitness in simply setting up opportunities for elderly people to join in some sort of regular activity. Even the very frail elderly have been shown to gain useful improvements in muscle strength from a short course of exercise. Exercise needs to be continued for the benefits to be maintained. Old people decondition just as fast as young people.

Many health centres and local authorities now have active programmes to encourage the over-50s population to take regular exercise. Among younger adults the aim is to get people to exercise at least three times a week for at least 20 minutes, doing something that makes them sweaty or out of breath. For older people, this intensity of exercise may not be feasible, and lower levels, such as brisk walking, may be better.

Stress management

Elderly people suffer from remarkable stresses: bereavement, poverty, and disability are obvious examples. Not surprisingly, when asked about their needs for prevention, stress management and relaxation are firm favourites. Successful group activities may involve a period of exercise followed by quiet relaxation achieved through breathing exercises, lying quietly, and listening to music. It is important to discuss the causes of stress and discover how people try to help themselves with difficulties. This can be a great source of group bonding.

General measures

To enjoy the benefits of exercise and to attend groups, some elderly people will need chiropody, help with arthritis and other sources of pain, and reliable transport. It is necessary to examine the nuts and bolts of preventive activities to ensure that it is feasible for elderly people to take an active part.

The location of activities is also important. No one likes to be surrounded by other similar people all the time. The geriatric ghettos of our day centres and senior citizens' clubs are unlikely to suit everyone. A health centre is an excellent base because it provides prevention for the whole population, not just the elderly. In other areas of health promotion, one-to-one contact with a health professional is one of the most effective means of achieving changes in behaviour and lifestyle. Opportunities for elderly people to discuss their health with primary health team staff must be developed in addition to group activities.

THE NEW GP CONTRACT

In the UK, general practitioners now have the responsibility for assessing all their patients over 75 years old once a year. This policy has been criticized because there is doubt about whether the time and energy invested will be rewarded by better health. However, the new contract does provide a good opportunity for health promotion, although this is not required under the terms of the contract.

Specifically, the contract requires that the following problems be looked for annually:

1. visual and hearing impairments;
2. immobility;
3. mental conditions (depression and dementia);
4. physical conditions (incontinence);
5. use of medications.

Identification of such problems is best viewed as tertiary prevention rather than primary prevention (see below).

SCREENING

Screening is the detection of disease at an early, pre-symptomatic stage before the patient would normally seek medical help. The best examples of screening are looking for high blood pressure, cancer of the breast and the cervix. There is good evidence to support screening for all three of these diseases, certainly up to the age of 75 years. However, policy does not accord with scientific evidence in this area, and many doctors and nurses do not routinely think it is worth including elderly people in such screening.

In practice, the benefits are likely to be at least as great, if not greater, among elderly than among young people. Why should this be? Taking high blood pressure as an example, many trials have now shown that treatment will reduce the risk of suffering a stroke by up to 75 per cent. Young adults have such a low risk of having a stroke, that even a very large reduction in risk will lead to only a handful of strokes prevented for many thousands of patients treated. Among older people the risk of stroke increases dramatically, so the same scale of treatment effect will lead to around 20–30 strokes prevented for every thousand patients treated.

The same arguments apply to cancer of the cervix and breast. The UK policy is not to routinely screen women over 65, provided they have an adequate previous screening history (at least three previous negative smears, the most recent in the last three years). This policy is not supported by evidence but is the view of an expert committee. Mammography screening has only recently been introduced in the UK with an upper age limit of 65 years. The evidence suggests that older women will probably benefit to the same extent as younger women, so again the policy is not informed by the scientific evidence and reflects ageist attitudes amongst policy makers. The best advice for women over 65 years is to request a cervical smear test every five years and mammography every three years, since the policy does not preclude patients seeking a test. By making regular demands of these services, elderly women will ensure that they are not ignored and may begin to influence policy makers.

CASE FINDING AND SURVEILLANCE

Case finding and surveillance are terms often used to describe the opportunistic detection of disease or problems. For example, case finding for high blood pressure is done by measuring the blood pressure of everyone turning up at the surgery. Screening, by contrast, would aim to measure all those people who do not turn up at the surgery. The costs and ethical aspects of the two approaches are quite different. Case finding, because it fits into the routine of practice, is relatively cheap and raises few ethical problems. Screening, because it has to seek out

everyone, is more expensive, and because the initiative is by the profession implies that the services are sufficiently good to deal with all the problems detected. For problems such as high blood pressure and cancer screening, a case finding approach is recommended.

TERTIARY PREVENTION

This is what many health professionals understand by 'screening' in old age. In fact it is detecting disease that is certainly symptomatic but largely *unrecognized or unreported*.

Elderly people are much more likely to have covert problems — incontinence of urine, depression and early dementia, immobility, falls, visual and hearing impairments — that are usually attributed to the ageing process, by both patients and health professionals. This is one of the reasons for the new UK general practitioner contract discussed above. It is hoped that detection of these problems will lead to improvement in the patient's physical, mental and social well-being. The evidence that sending a nurse or health visitor to look for such problems leads to improvement in health and well-being is extremely hard to find. Several trials have been conducted and resulted in equivocal results, suggesting that screening may save lives (but at the expense of greater disability in survivors), may save hospital admissions (in the days when there were more hospital beds), and may improve patients' morale (see Fig. 38.1).

There is little doubt that many patients welcome the attention and do wish to have an annual check-up. It is likely that such check-ups will reveal problems that require action, but it is less clear whether, as a society, we have the resources to meet such needs. In large part this will depend on the style of action wanted (or expected) by patients and offered by health professionals. Some evidence shows that elderly people are quite satisfied by their existing support systems, have tried several treatments for problems, and do not want any further action for their problems. This may, of course, be because past experience of health and social services has been so bad that expectations are very low.

It is likely that the new GP contract will lead to increased demands for hearing aids and ophthalmology clinic attendances, for referrals for social service home support, for investigation of incontinence. At

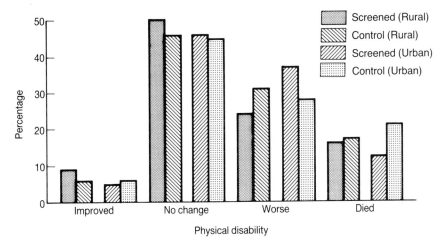

Figure 38.1 Results of a screening experiment in Wales, 1980/82 (Vetter, 1984)

present the skills of primary health care teams are not yet at a point where much of this work could be done within the health centre. Indeed, the time and special facilities required to assess a confused, incontinent or depressed elderly patient make it unlikely that it will ever be a major part of primary health care work.

The most optimistic view of check-ups for old people is that they give an excellent opportunity to review social networks and identify pre-crisis states. Much of the health service work with elderly people occurs around a 'crisis' that has been going on for many months, and usually years, without any sort of support for hard-pressed carers.

The most useful approach will be to focus upon those problems that patients want help with and are within the competence of the local services to solve. There is no reason why annual review of prescribing should not lead to fewer iatrogenic problems, why demented patients should not be referred to local support services and discussions on long-term care started and plans made and why increased numbers of frail dependent people should not be offered various types of respite care. The precise mix of what is possible will vary from area to area, depending on resources, and deficiencies will, of course, become much more apparent. Whether this will lead to increases in resources for elderly people is much more debatable, and will depend much more on younger elderly people exerting their political muscle.

Key points

- Elderly people are much more interested in modifying their lifestyles to achieve better health than professionals think.
- Primary prevention has much to offer old people: immunization (tetanus, influenza, pneumococcus); exercise; stress management; anti-smoking advice.
- Case finding for common problems (high blood pressure, breast and cervix cancer) in younger adults should be extended to the adults aged 65–75 years. Above this age the evidence of benefit is not available, but up to 75 years of age the evidence suggests that the cost–benefit ratio is greater than at younger ages.
- The 1990 GP contract requires GPs to offer a home visit to every person over 75 years to assess vision and hearing, mobility, mental state, physical condition, continence, and medications. It is hoped that this will lead to improvements in the physical, mental and social circumstances of old people. There is no evidence at present to support this notion.

FURTHER READING

Gray JAM. *Prevention in Old Age.* Churchill Livingstone, Edinburgh, 1985.

39 SEEING PATIENTS AT HOME

- Types of home visit
- Advantages of domiciliary consultation
- Disadvantages of domiciliary consultation
- Home visit before discharge

A unique feature of the National Health Service is the practice of home visiting by hospital specialists in health care of the elderly. Within the system there are two types of home visit.

1. *Domiciliary consultation*: the consultant visits to give a second opinion requested by a general practitioner (a fee is paid);
2. *Home assessment:* the visit is suggested by the hospital specialist to assess the need for admission (no fee is paid).

In the former case the GP is expected to be present if possible, and in the latter case the GP usually does not attend.

Soon after the start of the NHS when responsibility for the chronic sick was transferred to the hospital service the practice of hospital specialist visiting (often accompanied by a social worker) to assess urgency of admission was commenced. In the specialty of health care of the elderly this pre-admission assessment was often forced owing to the lack of resources, especially acute hospital beds. Such visiting continues to form the cornerstone of a few departments in the country. In most units such

assessment visits have ceased although paid domiciliary consultations continue.

ADVANTAGES OF DOMICILIARY CONSULTATION

Second opinion at home

One advantage of the system is that the GP can request a second opinion in the patient's home. Sometimes social conditions make it difficult to specify which problems should be regarded as contributing to the need for admission. A domiciliary consultation from a consultant is often requested in these circumstances.

History-taking

There can be considerable advantages gained from seeing elderly people in their own homes. In hospital history-taking may be difficult because of deafness, poor memory, speech impairment or confusional states. At home it is usually possible to obtain a more accurate and comprehensive history from a relative or neighbour who may well not be present in the outpatient department or on admission. The true problems are often identified in this way.

Educational value

Joint visiting (when GP and hospital specialist meet at the patient's home) can often benefit both; the GP being informed of new and previously hospital-based therapies and the specialist having the totality of the patient's dilemma illuminated by the GP's unique longitudinal information. Many hospital specialists take students on the domiciliary consultation to add to their insights into the complexities of health care in this age group.

Alternatives to admission

After the visit, advice can be given concerning the diagnosis(es), the likely chain of events and possible intervention using physical or drug remedies. A particular style of living may need to be adopted temporarily (e.g. one-room living with commode) and/or the use of Social Services may then prevent a hospital admission. Some districts have 'hospital at home' schemes or other forms of extra care provision to help keep a person in the community. Occasionally simple ideas may aid carers — such as advice on lifting, or the provision of continence aids.

Knowledge of home circumstances

This aspect of home visiting may be the most important but its true value only appreciated later (following a subsequent admission when discharge plans need to be made). This insight by clinicians is unique. Note can be taken of accident hazards (difficult stairs, worn or loose carpeting, low furniture, uneven low beds or an outside lavatory). There may be signs of self-neglect or neglect of the home with inadequate heating, poor food store provision and the non-functioning of the bath and toilet. This information is of great value when planning an eventual discharge as these problems stay vividly in the mind when seen at home prior to admission.

Domiciliary visits have been known to be conducted through the letterbox and the cause of immobility diagnosed through the kitchen window. Official identification is essential.

Consultation with relatives

Relatives or carers may be approaching exhaustion or already totally 'burnt out'. Some severely stressed relatives expect (even demand) that the visiting doctor take the patient away immediately even if the patient's condition does not warrant this. However, if help is needed it is essential that this is given as soon as possible and in some cases immediately (admission, day-hospital, etc.). This promptness helps later when discharge is contemplated and relatives/carers then know that they will be supported in their care-giving role.

Admission should be arranged before the situation becomes so critical that the relatives/carers feel that they cannot perform that role again. During the domiciliary visit time should be allocated to listen to the carer's point of view and then to outline the planned policy of treatment, rehabilitation and eventual discharge. In this way the carer realizes that admission to hospital will not be permanent.

Terminal care

Sometimes a visit reveals that a person is terminally ill and that death will be soon or inevitable. In these circumstances transfer to hospital may not be justified and a better course of action is to discuss the prognosis frankly with the relatives (and usually with the patient if the circumstances are appropriate), giving time to listen to the worries of all concerned. Then by liaising with the GP it is usually possible to arrange for extra home support (district/'Macmillan' nursing) by day and night.

Insight into social networks

Through domiciliary visiting one becomes aware of the unique nature of the individual's social network. One comes to realize that there is no such thing as total independence, for each of us is dependent upon others. Rather one realizes that there is relative acceptance and tolerance. The medical diseases may be the same but the social networks are not and a plan of management that ignores this holistic approach is doomed to failure.

DISADVANTAGES OF DOMICILIARY CONSULTATION

Conflict

Rarely conflict may arise when there is a difference of opinion as to treatment options between GP, consultant and carer.

Delay in gaining treatment

Most visits should be carried out within about 24 hours of the request unless otherwise specified. If a change in treatment results or admission is needed the domiciliary consultation may lead to an extra delay. This can be lessened by the specialist and GP meeting on the visit (as is theoretically required) or by the use of the telephone once the assessment is over. However, ill-health does not present classically in the elderly, and while a 'classic' urgent presentation may result in a quick admission, a slower 'gone off their legs' or 'failure to thrive' may be presented as a 'social problem' with inherent delays along the way. Also it should not be forgotten that in rural areas (and in heavily congested inner cities) considerable amounts of consultant time can be spent in travelling.

Lack of diagnostic facilities

Poor home circumstances can mean that the patient is not examined fully and an outpatient or day hospital appointment needs to be arranged so that a thorough clinical examination can be undertaken. In addition, apart from clinical acumen the investigations that are possible are obviously more limited than when the person is seen at the hospital. Some doctors consider that these clinical disadvantages are sufficient to make home visiting impracticable whilst others think the benefits far outweigh the disadvantages.

HOME VISIT BEFORE DISCHARGE

A *home visit* is also the term used when hospital-based therapists (OT, physio) accompany a patient home for a few hours to assess all of the discharge needs. Other professionals (e.g. the social worker) may also be present as well as carers. This visit can assess the patient's stamina, physical and mental skills as well as the home circumstances (furniture, stairs, hazards). It is a good opportunity to meet relatives and neighbours who may strongly express their concerns. Tasks may be set and their successful completion reassure both therapists and carers. The patient may do very well on the visit and concerns be allayed. However, there may be further rehabilitation needs identified or structural alterations deemed necessary. The need for formal and informal carer input can be assessed and a discharge plan identified with agreement that a certain level of input (from whatever source) can actually be achieved.

Home visits on the day of hospital discharge should be discouraged. Unexpected problems may arise and therapists and carers may be put under extra stress to prevent a readmission to hospital. In difficult circumstances a 'trial' at home is arranged with the appropriate professional calling in to the patient's home to check on progress. In ideal circumstances a post-discharge 'check' home visit can be used to allay fears and monitor the peri-discharge process.

Key points

- Domiciliary consultations are requested by the GP and are for the purpose of giving a second opinion on a patient's diagnosis and/or management. They are not used to assess the need or priority for admission to hospital.
- Advantages of domiciliary consultations are: ease of obtaining a second opinion; a more accurate and comprehensive history may be obtained; educational value; may be an alternative to hospital admission; knowledge of home circumstances may be valuable in management; relatives may be seen more easily and insights gained into social network.
- Disadvantages of domiciliary consultations are: conflicts may arise between doctors, patient and family; delay in treatment may occur; there is a lack of diagnostic equipment available.
- Home visits may be done prior to discharge from hospital by various members of the ward team. This allows better assessment of the patient's needs on discharge.

FURTHER READING

Arcand M, Williamson J. An evaluation of home visiting of patients by physicians in geriatric medicine. *Br Med J* 1981; **283**:718–720.

Dowie R. National trends in domiciliary consultations. *Br Med J* 1983; **286**:819–822.

Littlejohns PC. Domiciliary consultations — who benefits? *J R Coll Gen Pract* 1986; **36**:313–315.

Mulley G. Domiciliary visits. *Br Med J* 1988; **296**:515.

40 THE ELDERLY PATIENT IN ACCIDENT & EMERGENCY

- The problem
- The medical diagnosis
- The social set-up
- Appropriate referral
- Returning home
- Local authority Part 3 admission
- Admission to hospital

Elderly people form a disproportionately large part of the work of the A&E departments which have yet to come to terms with their needs. It is now accepted that children should be seen in a separate part of the A&E department, that special training and consideration of both child and parents are needed to ensure high standards of practice. The same could be said of elderly people, but it will take much effort to persuade A&E departments of the wisdom of treating elderly patients as a priority.

THE PROBLEM

The problem is all too familiar: an elderly woman arrives by ambulance in a confused state, with a daughter who is upset having found her mother on the floor at the bottom of the stairs. The patient does not seem too bad, and nothing medical seems to be wrong. The daughter then tells the casualty officer that it is obvious that her mother cannot go back home tonight.

In these circumstances, the casualty officer is forced into a role of gatekeeper to a scarce resource — a hospital bed for an elderly, confused woman. A confrontation seems likely, which makes the casualty officer annoyed, so he appears aggressive. There are no geriatric beds, the last one was filled hours ago, and the medical take-in team do not like 'confused grannies'. The patient lives alone, and was not coping too well anyway according to the daughter. Things really came to a head when the next door neighbour was taken ill and went into hospital the previous week.

The problem is the usual undifferentiated mix of medical problems, social support mechanisms, and immediate placement — or disposal from A&E. Unfortunately, it is very easy to muddle these different aspects of the case, and thus fail to come to the correct solutions. The crucial first step is to tackle each dimension of the problem separately, before making a judgement. This does of course take time, and requires just the same patience and tact as dealing with a two-year old who may or may not be seriously ill.

THE MEDICAL DIAGNOSIS

Elderly patients present non-specifically (just like children), and multiple pathology is frequent. It is usually necessary to rule out various common diseases systematically (see Table 40.1).

Table 40.1 Questions the house officer should ask before sending an elderly patient home from A&E

History
Is the patient normally well?
Is the patient on any medication?
Is the patient normally rational?

Examination

General
Is the patient confused?
Is the patient pyrexial or cold?
Is there a tachycardia?
Is the patient dehydrated?

Chest
Is there evidence of respiratory distress (count the rate)?
Is there evidence of pneumonia?

Heart
Is there evidence of heart failure?
Is there postural hypotension?
Has the patient had a silent heart attack?

Neuro/locomotor
Does the patient have evidence of a stroke?
Can the patient walk?
Could the patient have a hip fracture?

Miscellaneous
Could it be a urinary tract infection?
Could it be an overdose?
Is there blood on rectal examination?

Investigations

Urea and electrolytes:	Electrolyte disturbance?
Chest X-ray:	Signs of pneumonia or heart failure?
Urine/MSU:	Blood and/or pus cells?
ECG:	Acute infarct or dysrhythmia?
Blood sugar:	Diabetes or hypoglycaemia?

All this may seem 'over the top' to the busy casualty officer with plenty of 'real' patients to see. However, it is extremely rare for such a medical diagnostic approach to be negative, and even rarer for presentation at A&E to be precipitated for purely social reasons. If a social crisis does appear to be the prime cause of attendance, it is always worth asking whether it was precipitated by an acute medical problem. Often that problem will turn out to be confusion.

Assessing the confused elderly patient is not easy without some history. The crucial point to decide is whether the confusion is of recent and acute onset, or whether the patient has been gradually deteriorating for a period of many months or years. The patient will never be able to tell this piece of information to the doctor, so some other witness must be found. This may involve telephoning relatives, neighbours, the community psychiatric service, social services, or the family doctor.

It is simply negligent to state that, owing to the person's confusion, no history or examination could be done. It is also surprising how information can be obtained if it is asked for — even old hospital records can be found and may contain much needed clues to the present problem.

A side-effect of fully investigating elderly people in A&E is that it takes time. A&E trolleys are hard, with mattresses that are far too thin to protect elderly patients' skin. Pressure sores frequently have their origin in the A&E department, but are too often blamed on the receiving admission ward. Pressure sore prevention measures are as much the responsibility of A&E staff as any other hospital department, and appropriate mattresses should be used for immobile elderly patients.

THE SOCIAL SET-UP

Elderly people live within social networks, just like anyone else. Sometimes these networks are very supportive, sometimes they are as frail as the elderly patient. It is necessary to make enquiries about social networks, to work out who are the key people in this particular patient's life, the services received, the type of home lived in. This background information is essential in making a decision about referral. If the patient is to go home, the A&E department has a responsibility for knowing what 'home' means (e.g. outside lavatory, no central heating, and no home care services).

Often, local social service departments run 'good neighbour' schemes, or frail elderly schemes to help with the acute support of patients who do not require hospital admission but are unable to look after themselves for relatively short periods of time. It is only by contacting local social services that such information can be obtained. Contact should be made regardless of the expected outcome (going home or admission). In the latter case services may have to be cancelled, and considerable anxiety (and broken down doors) can be avoided by telling a home help that her client is in hospital. The task may of course be delegated to a social work assistant attached to the A&E department.

Communication with the family doctor is also of vital importance. The family doctor may have information about diagnoses, medication, and if the patient is going home, must be informed so that the patient can be reviewed the following day. Formal methods of communication between A&E and family doctors are frequently poor, and should not be relied upon for frail elderly patients. The responsibility rests with the casualty officer to contact family doctors by phone at the end of the shift.

APPROPRIATE REFERRAL

A proper medical assessment, having been made, it is usually clear what the next steps must be. Admission to an acute medical ward is not always necessary, although this is often seen as the easiest way out of a confrontation, and avoids the need for collecting so much information. It is often not in the patient's interests to be admitted to hospital unless medically essential. Typically, a request is made to admit an elderly patient with a toxic confusional state. In practice the diagnosis frequently turns out to be a dementia syndrome that is obvious after the first telephone call has been made to a relative.

RETURNING HOME

It is often necessary to discuss return home with friends and relatives, who may feel that they have 'done their duty', and that they no longer wish to provide care and support for a frail elderly friend. Such feelings are understandable and need to be talked through. Often a compromise can be reached enabling the elderly patient to return to their own home, while a more durable plan is built up with the help of the appropriate hospital and community services. Indeed, if the problem has been precipitated by an acute illness, it is likely that things will return to normal within a few days. Such negotiation is not normally part of the training of casualty officers, and is probably best done by specialists in health care of the elderly.

LOCAL AUTHORITY PART 3 ADMISSION

All social service departments have an on-call duty officer around the clock, and emergency places are available in Part 3 old people's homes. These are intended for genuine social emergencies (e.g. the death, or admission to hospital, of a carer). The patient has to be reasonably well: mobile, continent, and needing only minimal help in activities of daily living.

ADMISSION TO HOSPITAL

If the medical problem is surgical or orthopaedic this does not usually present any difficulties. With medical problems there can be confusion over referral to geriatricians or physicians. Most hospitals now have an acute medical take-in policy which aims to clarify relationships between the two specialties (see Chapter 35). Policies are either integrated with general medicine or age-related (e.g. over 75 years). It is important to know which system operates in the district, so that time is not wasted contacting the wrong service. However, a degree of patience is needed, because whatever the policy, beds are never empty when they are needed, and it will always take at least one more phone call than expected to admit an elderly patient from A&E. Casualty officers who have done a sensible job of making a diagnosis, of finding out about the social set-up, and working out an appropriate plan should have little need to play 'pass the parcel' with their elderly patients. It should be obvious where they need to go.

A further trap for the unwary is catchment areas. Most geriatric and psychiatric services admit only those people living in the district, and do not take admissions from out of the district. This is largely because of resource constraints and service contracts, rather than bloody-mindedness!

Key points

- An elderly patient presenting to A&E requires a thorough assessment. Corners cannot be cut, and obtaining background history is essential.
- Casualty officers should have a standard framework for their enquiries to aid ruling in or out common problems such as infection, stroke, and heart failure.

- Social services do provide help for genuine social emergencies, but are not a dumping ground for people with undifferentiated problems.
- A&E departments should be aware of the geriatric and general medicine admission policies, and local catchment areas. Provided the patient has been properly evaluated, discharge from A&E is seldom a problem.
- Old people are vulnerable to developing pressure sores while waiting in A&E. All beds and trolleys for immobile old people should have adequate pressure relieving devices.

FURTHER READING

Dove AF, Dave SH. Elderly patients in the Accident Department and their problems. *Br Med J* 1986; **292**:807–809.

41 DISCHARGE FROM HOSPITAL

- Discharge planning
- Informing the GP
- The first 48 hours
- Checklist

During a patient's stay in hospital the aim is to get him or her well enough to leave and return home. If at the end of the treatment the discharge is unplanned the effect is to undo all that has been achieved and possibly cause a traumatic period at home or a readmission. This can severely undermine a patient's confidence in their ability to manage ever again.

DISCHARGE PLANNING

This begins on the day of admission and is based on a full physical, mental and social assessment. It is vitally important to ascertain the usual lifestyle *prior* to admission (and prior to acute illness). This information may need to be obtained from many sources especially when dealing with a confused patient. In the course of the total assessment, answers should be obtained to the questions in Table 41.1.

Careful interviewing technique is essential to avoid such devastating comments to carers as: 'Your mother must never be left alone again.' Such thoughtless remarks can ruin lives.

Set realistic goals

A picture of a patient's lifestyle prior to admission is formed taking into account their present physical and mental state, and rehabilitation targets can be set. These must be realistic; a patient who has not walked for five years but managed at home is unlikely to walk again simply because of an admission to hospital. Discharge planning requires teamwork, but central to

Table 41.1 Discharge planning: Questions to ask

1.	Type and position of accommodation?
2.	Owner occupied or rented accommodation?
3.	How many floors and stairs?
4.	Position of bathroom and toilets?
5.	Does the person live alone, with family or with others?
6.	Visits/trips out? Frequency?
7.	Shopping, clubs, church, social activities?
8.	Visitors? Frequency?
9.	Relative/neighbour support?
10.	Social Service/health service visits?
11.	Family/carer perception of clients well-being?
12.	Client's perception of own well-being?
13.	What does the client *want* on return home?

this theme is that the patient understands and agrees to what everyone is trying to achieve.

Home assessment

It may be necessary for the occupational therapist or physiotherapist to undertake a home visit prior to discharge. Only then will the team know what difficulties the patient still has (if any) and what extra help will be necessary. The visit must be explained and agreed with the patient and often the carers, who in certain circumstances find this a threatening situation (e.g. the potential discharge of a patient whose carers consider should be 'in care'). All aspects of daily living can be assessed as well as orientation within the home surroundings — many chronically confused people perform badly in hospital but do well when in their own home.

Some aids and adaptations may take many weeks to organize and a priority list should be made (essential, advisable, non-urgent, etc.). Adjustments should be made only with the patient's agreement that they will be helpful.

During the visit the opportunity can be taken to talk to neighbours. It may be possible to find out what help, if any, they are prepared to give, but it is important that unreasonable demands are not placed upon them and that they should know where to turn to for help.

Following the visit it may be necessary for the team to meet with the patient and family/carers and decide on what needs to be organized, especially the role of new or extra help. The social worker usually plays a key role in discharge planning (with the ward nursing staff) and is often the patients' advocate, aware of their attitudes to the discharge and the future.

Timing and coordination

A crucial decision is the day of discharge. It is irresponsible to discharge an elderly person living alone and dependent on services on a Friday. A Monday discharge means that the patient has the benefit of five days of help and support prior to the weekend. On the other hand a weekend discharge is often best when the person is returning home to relatives/carers/neighbours who otherwise work and who provide a lot of input. Patients and relatives should have the telephone numbers and addresses (and even the names) of the support staff who are going to visit them at home (e.g. district nurses, bath assistants, home help, meals on wheels organizer). If there is then a problem the relevant person or organization can be contacted directly with minimal delay. Many services now insist on assessment visits so that the services themselves decide with the client what they need and how it will be provided. This may mean some degree of uncertainty prior to discharge as patient and carer can only be told that a service has been applied for. Some services are under severe strain in certain areas and the hospital staff should not imply to patient or carer that a service is automatic. It is far better to let the service manager discuss the situation with the client/carer, and if it is a vital service necessary for discharge one should endeavour to arrange a meeting of the relevant parties on the ward. Early referral to any service is essential. In difficult circumstances a case conference may prove necessary.

Prior to discharge any drug regimen should be made as simple as possible, and doctors, nurses and pharmacist should ensure either that the patient is safely self-medicating or that suitable alternatives are made. All patients should be issued with a drug card stating the drugs being taken, the dose and reason for prescribing (colour and shape can be useful). Any changes in medication must be noted on the card by the patient's GP.

INFORMING THE GENERAL PRACTITIONER

Close cooperation and communication between the hospital doctors and the patient's GP is essential. Ideally the GP takes part in discussions prior to discharge (especially in difficult cases). Failing this the GP should be contacted on the day before discharge by telephone, with full information regarding the diagnosis, treatment and medication as well as the support service arrangements and follow-up. This information should also be sent out by post in a short letter unless the discharge summary (a brief document containing only essential information) is sent within 24 hours of discharge (see Fig. 41.1). Outpatient or day hospital attendance should be made in advance and the patient, carer and GP informed.

```
┌─────────────────────────────────────────────────────────────────┐
│ DISCHARGE SUMMARY                                                 │
│                                                                   │
│                                                                   │
├───────────────────────┬─────────────────────┬───────────────────┤
│ Name:                 │ Consultant:         │ GP:               │
│ Address:              │ Admitted:           │ Address:          │
│                       │ Discharged:         │                   │
│                       │ Ward:               │                   │
│ DoB:                  │ Discharge address:  │ Dictated:         │
│ Hosp number:          │                     │ Typed:            │
├───────────────────────┴─────────────────────┴───────────────────┤
│ PROBLEMS                       ACTION                            │
│                                                                  │
│                                                                  │
│                                                                  │
│                                                                  │
├──────────────────────────────────────────────────────────────────┤
│ PRESENTATION                                                      │
├──────────────────────────────────────────────────────────────────┤
│ DRUGS                                                             │
│ Admission           Discharge           Allergies               │
│                                                                  │
│                                                                  │
│ Drug card(s)                                                     │
├──────────────────────────────────────────────────────────────────┤
│ DOMICILE                    CARER                               │
│                                                                  │
├──────────────────────────────────────────────────────────────────┤
│ FUNCTION                                                         │
│ Previous            Discharge           Mental                  │
│                                         Test                    │
│                                                                  │
├──────────────────────────────────────────────────────────────────┤
│ SUPPORT SERVICES                                                 │
│ Previous                    Discharge:                          │
│ Service     Frequency       Service        Frequency           │
│                                                                  │
├──────────────────────────────────────────────────────────────────┤
│ FUTURE PLANS                                                     │
│ Follow up                       Points for follow-up            │
│ Long-term plans                                                 │
├──────────────────────────────────────────────────────────────────┤
│ INFORMATION GIVEN                                                │
│                                                                  │
│ SHO name:          Bleep number:     Signed ................... │
└──────────────────────────────────────────────────────────────────┘
```

Figure 41.1 Discharge summary

THE FIRST 48 HOURS

This is the crucial period for many elderly people discharged from hospital. Some units have discharge teams (social workers or health visitors) who monitor the person's progress and report back. They are also available for any crises that may occur. 'Social' crises invariably arise as a result of an underlying medical issue and the GP with the information from the recent admission will be able to decide what action needs to be taken. Occasionally problems arise owing to carer 'breakdown'. These can be minimized by adequate pre-discharge planning and counselling. Pre-discharge arrangements should ensure that services are organized. In the event of problems the patient/carer must know where to obtain the relevant and specific explanation. Unavoidable readmissions do occur often owing to new illness episodes, unrecognized illness 'brewing' during discharge planning or unexpected accidents (falls, etc.). These should become learning exercises and form a specific part of a unit's *auditing* process. Avoidable readmissions are time-consuming, wasteful of resources and an unpleasant upheaval for the person concerned.

CHECKLIST

Attention must be paid to the small but essential items: food at home, keys, home security (during admission and post-discharge), adequate heating, aids fitted/delivered, spectacles/hearing aids/teeth *return* home with the patient, transport booked (the correct type), and follow-up arrangements made.

It is important to find out if the patient *wants* to return home. Many patients have anxieties but in spite of these they wish to be at home. For a few, however, going home is an appalling prospect. They consider it lonely, often frightening and either wish to stay in hospital or move to what they consider to be more suitable accommodation. The patient may not volunteer this but then perform unexpectedly badly on a pre-discharge visit. The patient should be counselled and as many anxieties as possible worked through. Except in the most difficult cases, however, the person usually has to return home while alternative arrangements are being made. For a few their anxieties are so great that despite performing well on the ward the discharge fails dismally and readmission is necessary.

Table 41.2 gives a checklist of questions to answer prior to discharge.

Table 41.2 Questions to ask prior to discharge

1. Is the person really medically fit enough?
2. Does the patient want to go home?
3. Is the discharge date and timing suitable for the carers and services?
4. Have the points noted in the home visit been answered?
5. Have the ambulance (correct type) and services been ordered (usually 48 hours notice required)?
6. Is the drug regimen the simplest possible? Does the patient have a drug card?
7. Have the patient,carer and GP been told?
8. Has the follow-up (and its transport) been arranged?
9. Before the person leaves the ward, does he or she have all belongings, especially teeth, spectacles, hearing aids, keys, money and medication?

Given the motivation to stay at home, careful planning and a modicum of luck, the return home of the majority of patients will be a safe and happy event.

Key points

- Discharge planning begins on admission with a full assessment.
- Realistic goals help patient morale.
- A home visit/assessment is necessary for many elderly patients, especially if there are team or carer doubts concerning the patient's ability.
- Day of discharge is important: early in the week is best for patients being supported by services, whereas a weekend may be more convenient for carers.
- Give the client and carers the names and telephone numbers of the services that have been booked.
- Liaise with the GP *prior* to discharge in difficult cases.
- Review and audit readmissions; they provide good learning exercises.
- Develop a discharge checklist.

FURTHER READING

Gay P, Pitkeathley J. *When I Went Home: A Study of Patients Discharged from Hospital*. King Edward's Hospital Fund for London, Pitman Press, Bath, 1979.

Simpson PJE, Levitt R. *Going Home: A Guide for Helping the Patient on Leaving Hospital*. Churchill Livingstone, Edinburgh, 1981.

42 THE ROLES OF THE TEAM MEMBERS

- Carers
- Chaplains
- Chiropodists
- Clinical psychologists
- Community psychiatric nurses
- Continence advisers
- Dentists
- Dietitians
- Doctors
- Hearing therapists
- Health visitors
- Hospital management
- Nurses
- Occupational therapists
- Pharmacists
- Physiotherapists
- Social workers
- Speech therapists

CARERS

The holistic approach to patient care must involve the main carer in decision-making processes. Patient autonomy and independence must be respected but health care professionals ignore the wishes and needs of carers at their peril. The carers are an important source of detailed information during the hospital admission, especially in the mentally impaired client. They are essential elements in the pre-discharge discussion process and when it comes to talking about future patterns of care. The concepts of duty and burden can be difficult to disentangle from care, and carers often take their cue from professionals and hence often enter into a long-term commitment. These decisions may affect their own family, job and indeed health and hence advice should never be offered lightly in terms of 'your mother shouldn't be left alone', for example. Stress and caring is another controversial area. It is accepted that looking after a frail or demanding person can affect one's physical and psychological well-being. Lack of sleep affects everyone. However,the importance of this 'stress' in causing disease or physical abuse of the elderly person is debatable. The role of respite care in reducing stress is also not clear-cut, though in all these situations one should err on the side of providing as much help as possible to both carer and client.

Carers, as far as is ethically possible, need to be kept fully informed as to a person's disease state, progress and prognosis. Most patients want their carer to be as involved as they are though exceptions do occur and the cue for information giving must come from the patient. Disease states need to be explained fully, especially in 'chronic' conditions such as Parkinson's disease and Alzheimer's disease. Health care professionals need to have pamphlets or books at hand to recommend for further reading as very little information is retained in the formal setting of doctor/patient/carer interview or meeting.

Where possible the patient and carer should be offered referral to voluntary organizations specializing in the field concerned (e.g. the Parkinson's Disease Society, Alzheimer's Disease Society). These groups act as further information sources, research bases and as carer/patient support systems. They can offer very useful and practical advice on the particular difficulties of caring for someone with a certain condition.

Caring is not a new phenomenon but it is occurring under new circumstances for many people. In past generations the extended family assimilated grandparents, older aunts, uncles or cousins with disabilities because usually they lived under one roof and there were few alternatives to 'caring'. People were not better at the role in days gone by — the same stresses, frustrations and problems were present.

Now, however, we are in the situation of most children moving away from home and having considerable periods of freedom away from such commitments (often until late middle life). Alternatives are available, but society still looks (as does the recipient) to family — especially daughters — to fulfil the caring role when it is required. Altering work and home schedules after such long periods of time is undoubtedly very hard.

The amazing thing is that so many people continue to do it, be it due to love or a sense of duty. At any one time there are approximately six million people caring for others in the UK — a truly impressive statistic.

CHAPLAINS

In many hospitals the Chaplains (either hospital-based or from the local church) provide a multifaceted service. Their visits may be regular or occasional. They provide the hospital religious services for staff, patients and visitors but also offer the individual patient spiritual help. This may be supportive or in the form of counselling, or may be at a time of crisis such as severe illness, or impending death. As the community becomes more multicultural so do the religious needs of patients. Religious guidance for many faiths may be needed on a single ward, not only to serve the patients but also to advise the staff on the special needs and practices essential to that religion. The Chaplain may assume the role of visitor, friend or advocate and, where a close relationship exists, should be part of the team process. The role also extends into teaching so that medical, nursing and other students are exposed to the holistic approach involved in the best care of patients.

CHIROPODISTS

Despite the concern over mobility in the elderly, interest in their feet tends to be aroused only at a very late stage. Elderly patients may be unable to see their feet or reach them. They may have accepted painful feet as an ageing process. Indeed sensation in the feet may be impaired or even absent.

The chiropodist is not trained simply to trim nails and cut and attend to corns (which can themselves render a patient housebound and immobile, but are usually treated by a foot care assistant) but to diagnose and treat congenital and acquired foot problems. They recognize and treat the pedal manifestations of systemic disease — for example, the patient who presents with plantar perforating ulcers as a result of diabetic peripheral neuropathy, or the ischaemic changes seen in peripheral vascular disease, confirmed using clinical examination and Doppler studies. Diabetics, however, have a special need for regular chiropody.

The NHS chiropody service is available free to the following categories of patient:

1. men aged 65 and over;
2. women aged 60 and over;
3. expectant mothers;
4. mothers with children under one year old;

5. children under school-leaving age;
6. physically handicapped persons;
7. diabetic/medically at-risk persons on referral from a consultant.

Treatment and advice can be obtained from health centres, hospital outpatients, day hospitals and day centres (if mobile). If the patient is housebound a domiciliary visit can be made. Transport should be available to take a person to a community clinic or hospital.

In many parts of the country the number of chiropodists is totally inadequate, resulting in long waiting lists and practically no domiciliary service. Private clinics are increasing as the NHS service contracts. There is an urgent need to train more foot care assistants.

CLINICAL PSYCHOLOGISTS

The clinical psychologist is concerned with the application of psychology to clinical problems.

Advice

Assessment and diagnosis. There is evidence that psychometric evaluation is able to contribute to the differential diagnosis of functional and organic conditions in the elderly. It can help in the difficult discrimination between dementia and depressive pseudodementia. In addition, careful objective assessment can be helpful in the identification of cognitive and functional deficits and advising staff on rehabilitative procedures. Baselines can be established to guide staff in assessing rate of change and areas of improvement or deterioration.

Treatment and management. Treatments for the confused elderly are directed towards helping the individual to remain at home or in the community, and/or easing problems that create special difficulty within the home or institution. These may include treatments for specific behavioural problems which can prevent the elderly person from coping at home (e.g. incontinence, faecal smearing, wandering, noisy, aggressive or demanding behaviour).

Psychologists may be involved in working individually with patients (e.g. treating fears or phobias which may be incapacitating) and in employing psychological approaches to the treatment of depression. They may also be able to help with other problem behaviours which may be causing stress within the family. Such interventions are primarily concerned with counselling of — and in some cases training of — relatives and care staff.

Recent developments

Cognitive change and age. Developmental psychology has produced a broader knowledge concerning the effects of ageing and there is now increased insight into the complexities of cognitive change in the ageing brain. *There is no evidence of a simple progressive intellectual deterioration with increasing age.* Some of the behaviour changes reported in the elderly which have been attributed to intrinsic causes probably relate to environmental variables. Even in dementia where impairment of learning and memory function is established, the residual adaptive capability is being explored as are programmes which minimize the detrimental effects of learning deficits. In some dementing illnesses certain research conditions can produce near-normal levels of retention of previously learned material. The exact nature of the memory deficit is still a controversial issue. Clinical psychologists are interested in the practical implications, such as the management of the memory-impaired person, and devising memory aids etc.

Environmental factors. Knowledge of the impact of physical, environmental and social influences on behaviour, particularly in institutions, is also expanding. A wide range of environmental factors are involved including the role of the individualized environment, privacy, 'territorial' behaviour in maintaining a sense of personal identity, the effects of imposed 'social' space and the effects of staff attitudes. The effects of the physical environment are also becoming better understood. A reduction in light level may produce disorientation and falls, certain colour contrasts can produce misperception of depth — hence psychological interventions may involve environmental modification.

Institutional care. Despite some advances in institutional care, publications and official reports still indicate that the environment of old people in institutions is unstimulating, non-therapeutic and creative of high dependence in residents and low job satisfaction in staff. Greater involvement by psychologists has been requested in helping to develop a *therapeutic milieu* in wards and day hospitals and to develop programmes to help elderly people adjust to any failing functions. Evidence is accumulating to indicate that some deterioration is related to these environmental variables. Improvement may be seen following the use of:

1. *Stimulation and activity approaches.* The improved effects do not seem to continue after the outside stimulation has ceased.
2. *Reality orientation techniques.* These aim to reduce disorientation and maintain a sense of personal identity in a confused person by continually presenting him or her with information about their current reality, the day, date, time, name, place, etc. Several studies show improvement in intellectual, social and word behaviour with these techniques.
3. *Milieu approaches.* These aim to counteract social deterioration by attempting to provide patients with normal social roles (e.g. encouraging an elderly person to take as much responsibility for their care and management as possible, including the making of decisions concerning group living in old peoples homes). There are clinical reports of increased social cohesion and better self-care, increased responsiveness and reduced levels of incontinence using this approach. This is dependent to some extent on changes in attitudes of care staff.
4. *Behaviour therapy.* This is based on a careful analysis of the interaction between patient and his or her past and present environment to throw light on the process leading to disturbed behaviour. It can be used to try to improve various functional deficits, including problems in-self care, social interaction and disturbed behaviour which are often accepted as part of a chronic confusional state.

COMMUNITY PSYCHIATRIC NURSES

Community psychiatric nurses are qualified in psychiatric nursing and in addition often have general nursing training. They can work out of hospitals or be attached to community health centres. They assess, monitor and treat all aspects of psychiatric illness in the elderly, liaising with consultant psychiatrists. They have roles in education (client and carer) and supporting both groups in the community. They tend to specialize in some areas such as the management

and treatment of depressive disorders and the organic illnesses such as dementia. Some are involved in crisis intervention teams.

With an increasing number of mentally ill elderly patients requiring assessment and long-term support, the role of the community psychiatric nurse is one of great importance. By building up and liaising with the supportive social networks, and generating trust with both patients and carers, they are often able to maintain very mentally impaired people in the community.

CONTINENCE ADVISERS

Continence advisers are trained nurses with a special interest in the problems of both urinary and faecal incontinence in both sexes. They may be based either in hospital or in the community and can help in diagnosis and management. They work closely with other specialists, but usually initiate some investigations and refer on if necessary. Some advisers work out of specialist urodynamic units and hence are involved in conducting the more detailed investigations. They are experts in the management of incontinence and are able to give specific advice concerning all the continence aids available, their use by client or carer. Most will perform home visits for the very disabled and have knowledge of the services available in a community (laundry service, delivery of pads, etc.). In hospitals their help can be invaluable for the 'difficult' patient and in an education and teaching role. They need to be consulted early and certainly before discharge is contemplated. They are also a source of information on equipment such as the latest catheters, their different uses, cost and drawbacks. Their expertise is available to institutions such as Part 3 homes.

DENTISTS

Many elderly people have poor dental health and are handicapped by their dental condition. One dental investigation of elderly people living at home revealed:

1. 74 per cent were edentulous and many were wearing unsatisfactory dentures;
2. 59 per cent had lesions of the oral mucosa (mainly related to dentures);
3. 32 per cent complained of oral pain;

4. 30 per cent had difficulty in chewing their food;
5. 13 per cent felt embarrassed by their appearance, with dentures dropping during social contact.

Most dental treatment is carried out by general dental practitioners. Although people over 65 years take up a very small percentage of NHS courses of treatment, they pay a comparatively larger percentage of all the charges because their treatment often involves expensive items such as dentures. Most elderly people have very low expectations of their dental health and are not particularly demanding. This situation will change in the future as more people retain their natural teeth into old age and higher levels of care will be required.

Old people often face serious dental problems if they become ill. Poorly fitting dentures previously skillfully controlled may suddenly become unwearable. For the increasing number of dentate elderly with heavily restored mouths a high level of oral hygiene is required. If this is difficult to achieve because of severe illness, recurrent caries and progressive periodontal disease may necessitate removal of the teeth, leaving the patient edentulous with no previous denture-wearing experience.

In hospital a dentist may be available. Alternatively upon discharge the FHSA (Family Health Services Authority) can provide a list of dentists who may be able to help. Similarly if a person is housebound a dentist prepared to do domiciliary treatment may be contacted via the FHSA.

The Community Dental Service can treat disabled adults if they cannot arrange treatment from other sources.

Treatment

Initially an assessment is made and emergency treatment to relieve pain carried out. It is then necessary to make a long-term treatment plan which may include:

1. prevention of further dental disease by
   (a) scaling and polishing natural teeth
   (b) cleaning dentures
   (c) advice on oral hygiene and diet;
2. treatment by
   (a) restoration of teeth
   (b) provision of training appliances or new dentures.

New techniques such as palatal training devices (for use in dysphagic patients after stroke), or postgraduate dental advice from dentists specifically

Table 42.1 Risk factors for malnutrition

Social
Isolation — living alone
Recent bereavement
Few or no outside interests

Mental disturbance
Acute confusional states
Dementia syndromes
Depression

Physical disability
Immobile or housebound
Arthritis
Blind or partially sighted

Effects of drugs
Causing nausea — chemotherapy, digoxin, antituberculous drugs, antibiotics
Metabolic effects – anticonvulsants, aspirin/antiarthritic drugs, diuretics, anti-parkinsonian drugs (L-dopa)

Ignorance of nutrition
Widowers
Those only eating one meal per day
Pre-existing poor dietary habits
Obsessive ideas about food
Restricted variety of diet

Impaired appetite
Following illness
Due to other factors (e.g. social, mental, drugs)

Economic
Pensioner alone
Other high expenses (e.g. heating)
Poor knowledge leading to poor choice and unwise use of available money

Increased nutritional requirements
Bedrest
Pressure sores/chronic wounds
Pyrexia (esp. long-term)
Post trauma (e.g. fall/fracture)
Pre- and postoperatively

Poor dentition
No teeth
Ill fitting dentures
Decayed teeth
Poor gum condition

Regular use/abuse of laxatives

High alcohol intake
Replacing meals
No money for food
Impaired vitamin metabolism

Recent discharge from hospital

Institutionalization

trained to deal with the elderly and the very disabled, may be available in some areas.

It is strongly recommended that *all dentures are marked*. The loss of a denture can be extremely distressing and it is often impossible to produce satisfactory replacements. This is particularly important for patients in continuing care settings.

DIETITIANS

Formal studies have revealed what has always been suspected — there is a lot of malnutrition amongst the elderly. A high degree of suspicion is needed for diagnosis since most sufferers will have a subclinical picture. Florid scurvy is rare but does still exist. The role of the dietitian working with the elderly includes:

1. giving advice on nutrition in health and disease;
2. educating all people who work with the elderly to the need for a special understanding concerning the importance of nutrition;
3. the nutritional assessment and treatment of referred patients;
4. being a fully involved member of the multidisciplinary team.

Elderly patients requiring nutritional advice both in hospital and the community can be seen by the dietitian, usually following receipt of a referral form from the hospital doctor or general practitioner. A person may be at risk of malnutrition if he or she fulfils three or more of the conditions in Table 42.1.

One area of particular interest for the dietitian is the swallowing-impaired patient (most commonly seen after a stroke). The dietitian is involved from the outset with many other specialists (e.g. speech therapists) in assessing the swallow reflex and nutritional states and advising on the best regimen. Foods with varying consistency may need to be provided, or if nasogastric feeding is implemented (short or long term) the dietitian advises on the total body requirements.

It must not be assumed that people living within institutions will be well nourished. In one study 30 per cent of long-stay patients in hospital were at risk of scurvy. Others who did not go out in the sun were at risk of osteomalacia.

DOCTORS

Life is short and the art long; the occasion fleeting; the experience fallacious and the judgement difficult. The physician must not only be prepared to do what is right himself but also to make the perfect patient, the attendants and externals cooperate.   *Hippocrates—Aphorism 1*

Hospital doctors work in a hierarchical structure whereby ultimate responsibility for medical treatment resides with the consultant. Consultants expect the junior doctors to show that they have done their work to the best of their ability. They are expected to demonstrate that they have taken a first-class medical and social history (often needing details from relatives, carers and others), thoroughly examined the patient, written legible complete notes and requested the correct investigations. Junior staff are not expected to know everything, nor get everything right; but they are expected to demonstrate, firstly, that they have tried, and secondly that they are aware of their limitations. Doctors who do not give of their best let themselves, their patients and their colleagues down. Excuses for failure to write notes, obtain x-rays, etc., are unlikely to be accepted — remember that the consultant was once a junior too.

The biggest failing at all levels is medical arrogance. The belief that one knows it all is surely tested by regular post mortems. Always remember that the other non-medical members of the team know much more about their subject than the junior doctor. A useful tip is always ask the question *why?*. Identify the problems and try to group them together. Some doctors routinely use a problem list (e.g. problem-orientated medical records) or a disability profile to ensure that problems such as deafness and incontinence are not ignored. A biochemical profile is a useful addition to all notes. In acute wards a note should be written each day and on each occasion a procedure is carried out, drugs changed or a significant event has occurred (including summaries of conversations held with carers). In long-stay (continuing-care) wards a progress note should be written weekly.

The house physician is the 'key worker' for the majority of patients in the ward. He or she should know everything that is happening to the patients and is responsible for ensuring that other staff, the patients and carers know as well. This is the art of communication — it entails patience, good telephone skills and a pleasant manner often in the face of difficulty. The house physician is a collator of information. When talking to relatives junior doctors should collect relevant information but be careful about making value judgements or hasty statements like 'She should not be left alone' or 'She can never go home'. Sitting in with the consultant at difficult interviews (angry or anxious relatives) can be invaluable experience in learning how to handle these situations.

The house physician should prove a good link to the general practitioner in the primary health care team in the community. In all potentially difficult discharges (patient or relatives) the GP should be alerted prior to the discharge date. Similarly in cases where the GP should be forearmed with knowledge (recent diagnosis of carcinoma, unusual drugs, etc.) a telephone call is polite and valuable. Discharge letters and summaries should be *prompt*, *short* and *relevant* (see Chapter 41).

Requests for admission by general practitioners should not be questioned by junior doctors.

HEARING THERAPISTS

Hearing therapy is a relatively new discipline, introduced to provide more continuous and comprehensive help than was possible by issuing hearing aids alone. The therapist tries to help individuals with an *acquired* hearing loss make the most of their residual hearing, by teaching them to use every available auditory and visual clue, thus making it possible for them to live in a world that relies on language for communication with fewer anxieties.

The hearing therapist is concerned with rehabilitating the hearing-impaired person via programmes that include the following:

1. auditory training — encouraging a person to listen again through a hearing aid where speech is frequently distorted;
2. lipreading — teaching a person to watch facial expressions and lipshades to assist their understanding of speech;
3. help with a hearing aid — how to operate the controls and how to fit the earmould in the ear;
4. advice about environmental aids — television, telephone, doorbell etc.;
5. advice on how to cope with a hearing loss — counselling about the problems concerning home, work and social situations.

The disability of deafness

Society relies on the spoken word for exchanging ideas, commenting on events, expressing pleasure, relaying information and idle chatter, all of which add meaning to our lives. Failure to appreciate the spoken word can cause withdrawal from society (Beethoven being only one famous example). Most people perceive deafness as an inability to hear anything and

assume that the only way to communicate with the deaf person is to shout. It is a widely held view that with a hearing aid a deaf person will comprehend all spoken language and if the hearing aid is not worn then the person is being uncooperative, antisocial or even aggressive. The deaf person may be shunned and ignored. It is easier for people with good hearing to talk to someone who understands them rather than take the time and effort to communicate with the deaf person. Deafness affects one in three of the elderly and its onset can make a cheerful person become sullen, withdrawn, aggressive and over-anxious.

Recognizing the patient with hearing loss

1. Visual clues — leaning forwards, cupping hand behind the ear
2. Auditory clues — complaining about others mumbling, speaking loudly
3. Social history — door not answered, TV too loud, not attending family gatherings.

Action

1. Examine ears for wax.
2. Refer to ENT, for medical assessment of hearing.
3. Refer to ENT technician if hearing aid is malfunctioning.
4. Refer to hearing therapist.

Hearing aids

A person who wears a hearing aid successfully will feel more confident and less depressed and isolated. He will *not* receive clear speech automatically. A hearing aid amplifies all sounds equally; it does not correct impaired hearing but only amplifies sound. The controls on the hearing aid are difficult for the elderly to adjust and the earmould is difficult to fit.

How to assist the hearing impaired patient to communicate better

1. Attract the person's attention before you start to speak.
2. If possible exclude peripheral noise.
3. Speak slowly and clearly in a moderate voice.
4. Do not exaggerate lip movements.
5. Write down important facts.
6. Check if spectacles are worn.
7. Look at the patient when speaking with the light towards your face.

8. Sit at the same level as the patient.
9. Do not speak with your face covered.
10. Keep your hands still.
11. Check that the hearing aid is working.
12. Try an easi-com communicator.

HEALTH VISITORS

Hospital-based personnel are often vague as to the precise qualifications of a health visitor. They are all fully trained nurses or midwives with several years' experience followed by a one or two-year postgraduate diploma course at university or polytechnic. Health visitors are usually based in the community, either in child health clinics or sometimes within general practitioner's premises. Comparatively few specialize in the health care needs of the elderly.

There are four main functions of health visiting:

1. prevention of mental, physical or emotional ill-health;
2. early detection of ill-health and surveillance of high-risk groups;
3. recognition and identification of need and mobilization of appropriate resources where necessary;
4. provision of care: this includes support during times of stress, advice and guidance in case of illness and in the management of children

In the community the first priority is to children under five with a view to counselling the whole family. The basic role changes little on joining the team involved in health care of the elderly in that expertise in working with the whole family remains a very important part of the work. This is coupled with support of and liaison with the professional team.

The health visitor provides a link between the contrasting worlds of home and hospital. This is accomplished by visits to the home before, during and after admission and attendance at ward rounds for the sharing of knowledge. The health visitor can provide information and opinions on the following:

1. *Housing conditions* — will the patient be able to cope with their immediate environment or will changes need to be made.
2. *Relative support* — assessing the level of support carers will be able to provide following discharge.
3. *Neighbours' attitude* — often provides clues to the patient's inability to cope with emergencies.

In an ideal world (or at least an ideal NHS) every suitable elderly patient would have the benefit of a health visitor's assessment whilst in hospital and care after discharge (even if only for a short period in most cases). The peri-discharge period is fraught with complex difficulties and the expertise of a health visitor liaising between hospital and community can make the difference between a 'soft' and a 'hard' landing (or no landing at all and a readmission).

HOSPITAL MANAGEMENT

The first Griffiths Report on the Health Service recommended the introduction of a new management structure to improve communication, cut delays in decision making and to introduce the concept of budgets (cost-effectiveness) within a health care setting. Each health district gained a District General Manager (DGM) with specific Unit General Managers (UGMs) accountable to them. A new tier of finance managers was also incorporated and with the addition of medical and nursing representatives district management teams evolved.

This management structure has indeed revolutionized the running of most major hospitals and their community systems, though not without significant difficulties. The arrival of 'management' coincided with a widely held view that the NHS was significantly underfunded. Thus management decisions and indeed legal obligations to remain within budgets resulted in direct and indirect cuts in patient care (bed closures, longer waiting lists, etc.).

The management structure is now fully operational in all areas — inpatient, outpatient and community settings. Financial management is also in place with the aim of hospital and community sub-units having their own budgets and the autonomy of working within them. Management thus has significant responsibilities in information technology, aiming to provide the end user with the technical and budgetary details required to run their part of the organization effectively. Hence part of the new NHS world has been coming to terms with the new technology involved, computer skills, databases, software, budgetary skills.

This business-like approach to the NHS has manifested itself in the latest changes, that of purchase/provider separation. From 1 April 1991 hospitals and their community services become the *providers* of health care whereas the District Health Authorities, GPs (and hence patients) become the *purchasers*. Hospitals have to develop contracts concerning the type of health care they will endeavour to provide being acceptable to purchasers. In this way it is thought that the system will generate improvements via competition since purchasers will only place contracts where they will get high-quality value-for-money service.

Some hospitals have been allowed more freedom within this new system and have become Hospital (and in some cases associated community) Trusts. These trusts are still within the NHS and under the rules of purchaser/provider and contracting. They are able to raise capital independently (e.g. borrow money to fund new schemes) and have more autonomy in management decision making, hence improving their competitiveness. Little new money is available for direct care of patients and extra sums will be used to pay the management costs, an irony considering that before the reforms the NHS had the lowest administrative costs of any major health care system. The performance of the new NHS, and its 'market' approach, will be watched with great interest both in Britain and overseas. It is likely that an increased part of our gross national product will be directed to health care as the general public becomes more aware that the limitations in what they receive from the health service are a consequence of underfunding and not simply due to poor management.

NURSES

Nursing care in a ward for the elderly is different in that the greatest degree of caring often lies in consciously choosing to do less rather than more, in order to help patients regain independence. This can be difficult for nurses trained to do everything for their patients. Time is important; it is much easier (and quicker) to dress a patient than to wait while she takes the time to dress herself. Nurses have to allow the patient to dictate both tempo and routine.

There is emphasis on patient choice. If medication, therapy or any other form of treatment or care is refused this rejection must be considered sympathetically. The cause for refusal should be established and discussed. Occasionally it may be necessary to accept a refusal as being absolute. The object is not to force people to do what you want but, by encouragement and help, achieve the goal that they want themselves. Goals should be set within the patient's capabilities.

The dignity of the patient should be considered at all times. An apparently caring attitude of leaving a toilet door open to avoid accidents may be profoundly disturbing. If surveillance is necessary the nurse should be outside listening carefully with the patient enjoying the illusion of total privacy. Toilets and bathrooms should have call bells (clearly explained) so that a greater feeling of security is encouraged. Other important factors include drawing the curtains around when undressing, receiving treatment or being examined, and arranging for privacy when seeing relatives and friends.

Measures such as these enable the patient to maintain his or her sense of identity. This can be further fostered by encouraging patients and relatives to bring in familiar things such as family photographs. A sense of comfort and belonging follows and helps prevent the feelings of isolation. Visiting should be encouraged at all times of the day and even by special arrangement during the night. Visitors may be of all ages as usually none of the restrictions on children need apply (except in specific cases). Arrangements should be made for elderly friends to visit.

The nurse takes a great deal of responsibility and must therefore be involved in decision making. The aims, objectives and treatments must be clearly written down. The admitting nurse will complete the nursing profile or care plan where the care is planned in detail and updated as necessary. The aim is to show at a glance the diagnosis, progressive treatment and ultimate goal (e.g. to return home). In this way both the recording nurse and other nurses involved at a later date have a clear reminder of the pattern of care decided upon and any alterations in the patient's progress.

The Nursing Process

This is the name given to a more personalized method of patient care. It has two main themes:

1. A nurse has overall responsibility for a particular patient and develops a specific relationship with him/her.
2. Treatment is based on individual need.

The nurse involved with admitting the patient takes a history, fills in the nursing notes and prepares the care plan or nursing profile. One nurse is then given responsibility for the care and treatment of a certain number of patients during the shift. A student will be supervised by a trained member of staff. No nurse is required to administer treatment beyond the scope of their experience, but within these limitations the duties are carried out as indicated in the nursing profile. The order in which the treatments are carried out is determined as far as possible by the pattern of the patient's normal day when at home and by the availability of all members of the multidisciplinary team.

The second theme of the nursing process has four parts — assessment, planning, implementation and evaluation. Assessment includes the physical, mental and emotional state of the patient together with details of the home environment. Following this the individualized care plan is worked out based on specific needs and is then implemented. This is closely linked with the final part, evaluation, an on-going assessment from which comparisons are based on the patient's progress. The implementation involves not only the nurse but the whole of the multidisciplinary team.

OCCUPATIONAL THERAPIST

The occupational therapist provides a further cornerstone in the assessment, monitoring and advising on discharge and resettlement — providing for a better quality of life for elderly patients whether short, medium or long stay. The aims of occupational therapy are:

1. the assessment, maintenance/improvement of mental and physical function to enable the person to cope with the environment and to advise on resettlement if appropriate;
2. work with families to increase awareness of potential capabilities of the patient in hospital and in the community;
3. liaising with the multidisciplinary team and community services.

OTs work both in the hospital setting (with outreach services) and in the community (within Social Services). Early referral is essential. In many departments of health care of the elderly all patients are assessed (to find previously undiagnosed problems). OTs assess in terms of level of function (eating, dressing, coping in the kitchen) and provide reports on *activities of daily living* (ADL), home visits and suitability for old people's homes when specifically requested.

Role of the OT

1. Assessment and grading of level of function and suitability for home safety etc.
2. Improving/maintaining function (and general health) using graded tasks and activities to lessen fatigue and increase range of movements.
3. Restoring local function by use of remedial games, craft work, etc.
4. Helping the permanently disabled achieve maximum independence within the constraints of their disability.
5. Prophylactic measures (diversional therapy). The use of activities to stimulate patients mentally and physically to maintain a sense of well-being and encourage socialization. The activities should be purposeful and enjoyable.

Activities of daily living

These consist of the tasks undertaken daily to maintain levels of personal care. To the elderly person the ability to perform these tasks may mean the difference between returning home or not. Information obtained by questioning must be substantiated by observation (some people will exaggerate to get home and be unrealistic as to their true capabilities). Assessment includes ascertaining those activities that are deficient, evaluating the potential for improvement and deciding on a programme to achieve this potential.

Mobility. All mobility is considered and assessment of the environment (height of chairs, toilet, floor covering, tables, stairs — both in and out of hospital) is essential. Wheelchairs need skilled assessment to suit the needs of the patient and carers.

Eating and drinking. This is probably the area in which a very handicapped patient can attain independence. Special crockery and cutlery is available, as is expertise on arranging the dining area.

Toilet management. This is a crucial function for independence or resettlement. Practical solutions such as a hand rail or raised seat can sometimes cure incontinence. Commodes at night or chemical toilets can be invaluable but need ordering well in advance of discharge.

Personal hygiene and dressing. Assessment here should be as soon as possible after admission as increasing abilities can boost a patient's morale tremendously. Severe problems are often encountered but perseverance in dressing practice, the use of aids and self-care is essential.

Communication. Liaison with the other members of the team means that patients with communication difficulties can continue to receive therapy. Advice can be given on specific alarms or communication aids in the home.

Domestic tasks. Training must be combined with the knowledge of the patient's home circumstances. One must guard against the blanket provision of full services such as meals-on-wheels and home-help when the patient can cook and clean. Practice may be essential in some tasks, especially in those involving the kitchen (gas, boiling water). Remember that patients usually perform better in their own home. Many activities can be encouraged to increase general and local functioning — reading newspapers, gardening, games, etc. Some activities encourage social integration and will involve other staff members.

Home visits

Visits need organization (keys, access, joint visit, relatives or carers present) and then time to implement the findings. The assessment includes:

1. the patient's ability to cope with the accommodation and its furniture; its suitability in terms of the patient's disability (long and short term);
2. what (if any) aids/adaptations have been or need to be provided — essential or just useful;
3. the patient's attitude to the home environment, his motivation and wish to return home and cope;
4. the attitude of family/neighbours and support services to the patient.

Some units provide outpatient occupational therapy. If this is not possible, and continued therapy is thought necessary, it may be possible to refer patients to a day hospital or for them to receive domiciliary therapy.

PHARMACISTS

The role of drugs in the elderly — their dosage, interactions, side-effects and administration — is assuming increasing importance. The hospital pharmacist can advise on current medication and be involved in new prescribing. Possible drug interactions and the side-effects of medication can profoundly affect the success or failure of either a course of treatment or even necessitate a hospital admission. New formulations of drugs mean that more treatment options are open depending on individual circumstances. However, all these advances are often reflected in cost. The pharmacist can advise on the cost–benefit ratio so that the patient and hospital receive the best possible deal.

The pharmacist can also advise on the practical aspects of drug taking, fitting regimens to individuals and assessing the likelihood of compliance with self-medication trials, or the use of dosettes (small containers with a day's or week's worth of tablets). Most hospitals now operate their own drug policy, with doctors and pharmacists agreeing on a selected core of drugs for hospital use and the prescribing of drugs outside this core being by mutual agreement, with patient needs predominating.

Community pharmacists provide an advice and education service to many of their elderly customers. Surveys have shown that these pharmacists are often approached before GPs with medical problems. They often help with minor ailments and advise consultation with a doctor for the more serious complaints. They, like their hospital counterparts, can help explain treatment regimens, possible side-effects and the need for a course of drugs, often in a more relaxed environment leading to a better understanding by the patient.

PHYSIOTHERAPISTS

Physiotherapy remains one of the crucial points in the successful rehabilitation of elderly people by helping them to achieve maximum independence with minimal assistance. Most elderly people admitted to hospital are likely to need some form of physiotherapy and referral should be made at the earliest opportunity. The elderly benefit from prophylactic physiotherapy (preoperative breathing exercises, how to get up off the floor following a fall, etc.).

Methodology has three aspects:

1. reviewing the past history;
2. assessing the present problem;
3. planning a future programme.

Reviewing the past history often involves collating and reading the information gained from other professionals and asking specific therapy-orientated questions (layout of house, aids used, stairs/steps/slopes, garden, previous mobility).

Assessing the present problem involves seeing the patient at the earliest possible opportunity, often with other members of the multidisciplinary team. The assessment should begin with introductions and an explanation of the procedure involved. An experienced physiotherapist can quickly get an overall impression — the state of mood of the patient, their dress and general demeanour, communication problems, etc.

Table 42.2 A brief physical assessment

Raise arms above head	Balance in sitting
Hand grip/release	Reaching forwards
Lift feet	Sitting/standing
Right or left handed	Walking
Straighten knees	Use of aids
Lift knees	

The brief physical assessment is shown in Table 42.2. Continual assessment is made throughout the person's stay in hospital and modifications are made to accommodate improvements. A fuller assessment is shown in Table 42.3.

Table 42.3

Range of movement of all joints
Strength of muscle groups
Functional activities e.g. turning/moving in bed/lying/sitting over edge of bed. Bed to chair.
Dressing (liaise with OT)
Liaison with nursing staff over particular difficulties – transfers, i.e. chair to commode, sitting to standing.

Following assessment, the physiotherapist will plan a treatment programme, involving carers if appropriate. Goals will be set with the patients and family and progress will be monitored. The treatments used are eclectic (e.g. heat, ice, passive and active resisted movements, hydrotherapy, the Bobath technique — Table 42.4) and there is great variation between therapists in their approaches. Increasing effort is going into testing the effects of different treatments.

Table 42.4 The Bobath technique

A bilateral technique (i.e. not compensating the unaffected side)
Uses feedback, repetition and the full use of the affected side
Sensorimotor re-education to help decrease spasticity
The aim is to decrease spasticity to get normal movement patterns.

Home visits

A home visit *without* the patient can bring to light certain difficulties which can be simulated in hospital (e.g. different floor surfaces, deep steps). On home visits *with* the patient the physiotherapist takes note of any difficulties that occur with furniture, doorways and passages and can then provide assistance in planning a safer room and advise on sites for rails, ramps, etc. If relatives, friends or neighbours are going to have to assist a patient, then advice and technical guidance can be given to ease anxieties.

Future

All members of the team help in assessing and deciding when a patient has reached optimum mobility and function. This is the prime time for discharge, but the physiotherapist can be of continued help. Patients can be referred to the physiotherapy department or to the day hospital for continued help in maintaining them in the community. Domiciliary physiotherapy is a treatment service available to elderly people in their own homes (including sheltered accommodation) and old people's homes. Community physiotherapy is an assessment and advisory service — treatment can be arranged at either the physiotherapy department or the day hospital.

SOCIAL WORKERS

A social worker works with and on behalf of the client/patient in an advocacy role. The aims are to enable the client, through counselling, to cope with the problems and stress of daily living, and to obtain those services which are appropriate to their needs.

Social workers are employees of the local authority and most are based in the community, but there is an obligation to provide a hospital-based service because of the enormous needs of the clients there. Social workers mainly work in teams, often neighbourhood or 'patch' based. While the requirement is to serve all client groups, the reality is an overwhelming amount of child protection work, which is statutory. In many areas the elderly receive a poor, crisis service. In most large hospitals there are teams, one of which usually concentrates on the needs of the elderly and the elderly mentally ill.

Referrals

Referrals should provide basic personal information on the client (including contact phone numbers of relatives, wardens and other relevant people), state the aim of the referral (service provision or counselling role) and state whether the client is aware of the referral. Written requests are less common than the more informal approach during ward rounds or ward meetings. Indeed all patients should ideally be reviewed by a social worker who in an advocacy role may highlight certain dilemmas and change practice. Social workers can only *request* domiciliary services, they cannot demand them; hence patients should not be given absolute assurances of a certain level of support. These decisions are made by the relevant department or agency itself, guided by the social worker but usually after independent assessment. No two local authorities offer identical services, and the availability and cost to the client varies widely. Requests for services should be made as early as possible, because they are as crucial as the correct drugs and well-being of the patient if a successful discharge is the aim.

Social reports

The collation of general information on a patient's social/environmental background is not solely the responsibility of the social worker. A social report, however, is a detailed analysis of a patient's lifestyle involving, for example, relationships, attitudes, experiences and expectations. It cannot be compiled quickly and should not be requested unnecessarily.

Domiciliary care

In general, inner-city districts provide a higher level of resources than elsewhere (to compensate for the difficulties encountered — housing, isolation, etc.). In some areas domiciliary services will not start until a home assessment has been made (following discharge) and then the service may be limited initially. This can put a great strain on the client and carers. Home helps assist with basic household tasks. The term is gradually being replaced by home care, with some expansion of the role. Sometimes home care provides the only source of regular social contact and hence has a major role in monitoring how the client is managing. They can inform others in the social network of circumstances that may need attention or action.

Specialist teams (e.g. family aides) exist in some areas to provide an intensive level of support to selected clients in the first few days after discharge or following a crisis. They are designed to gradually withdraw and let the usual services take over responsibility. Some districts have domiciliary sitting services to allow relatives/carers a short break.

Meals-on-wheels

These were originally provided by the voluntary agency WRVS (Women's Royal Voluntary Service). In some areas voluntary groups have retained control of the service, but for most it is now administered by the local authority. Advantages include cost (most authorities charge clients a modest sum), the provision of one hot 'nutritious' meal a day, social contact and a basic requirement for the physically or mentally handicapped who could not prepare a meal. Disadvantages include timing (lunch may be delivered at 10.30am, with reheating problems), provision (up to five days per week may be arranged, seven days a week provision is scarce), quality ('Muck on trucks' is a verbatim quote!), and ethnic requirements (Jewish Kosher food is well established, but this is not the case for Halal meat for Moslems, and oriental tastes). Enormous sums of money are spent on meals-on-wheels, yet there is little research to indicate whether they are what the client wants or needs in terms of food provision.

Day care

The range of social activities is designed to meet needs for therapy, rehabilitation, assessment, stimulation and respite for family/carer.

Luncheon clubs are mainly used by the active elderly in their immediate neighbourhood. They provide inexpensive meals and act as social centres.

Day centres cater for a mixed client group but usually can manage the less active, and transport is arranged. They offer a wide variety of activities to cater for most tastes. The larger establishments may have a social worker, OT and physiotherapist attached part-time.

The very frail (though not in need of nursing attention) may also attend a day centre, but often their day care is within a residential unit, or attached to one. Some units are open seven days a week and offer a means of assessing suitability for alternative care as well as providing rehabilitation.

Sheltered housing

This is specifically designed accommodation for elderly people, usually in the form of flats. There is the added security of a warden to help in an emergency. Sheltered housing varies in its complexity, from accommodation for the very frail with a warden calling twice a day, to units where tenants are expected to be virtually independent and where the warden is not 'on site' and has periods 'off' altogether. Each Social Service housing department should have someone informed about the local availability and provision of warden help.

Residential homes

The term 'Part 3' home arises from that numbered section of the National Assistance Act 1948 which states that it is the duty of every local authority to provide 'residential accommodation for persons who, by reason of age, infirmity or other circumstances, are in need of care and attention which is not otherwise available to them'. However, this is qualified by the statement that such accommodation should not provide 'services of a kind normally provided only on admission to a hospital'; that is, it is not designed to offer nursing care. Residents are means tested and if possible pay for their care at the going rate. Once resident most of their pension is taken to offset the cost. On admission they are expected (and may be rejected if not) to be mobile with or without aids, able to attend to basic daily needs with the minimum amount of supervision (i.e. dress and be continent), and capable of adjusting to living in a communal environment. The elderly mentally infirm may be accommodated in special units (EMI homes) or placed in the ordinary units. Each local authority has its own system of either integration or separation.

Residential homes have historically been staffed at levels consistent with this concept of frail but independent. The reality of the last 10 years, however, has been that the homes are inundated with increasingly more frail people in need of higher and higher levels of care. Numerous studies have shown that in most residential homes the majority of residents are both confused and incontinent. Staffing levels are too low and morale is down, accompanied by poor pay and a distinct lack of training. Despite this some homes are places where you would happily entrust a loved one (a good test) whilst others conform to Victorian workhouse descriptions.

Private care

The 1980s saw a government-led explosion in the private sector, both residential and nursing home. Through Department of Social Security (DSS) funding, tens of thousands of people are now in private institutions. Choice was argued as a reason — to be nearer relatives, pay for added luxuries, type of home, etc. Private homes can provide a wider range of choice, from rest homes with minimal care to nursing homes with intensive nursing help. However, the harsh financial reality is that most homes are finding it difficult to stay in business on DSS rates alone (let alone provide 'extras'), and hence the financial gap has to be met either by the resident or the relatives. In addition the homes have minimal official supervision, even though they have to be registered, and the resident has few legal rights. These issues should be widely and openly explored *before* a person goes in. The closure of hospital beds and local authority Part 3 places has increasingly forced many districts to use the private sector. Indeed some areas no longer have a NHS or local authority controlled long-stay resource. The implications of these changes alongside the other monumental changes in the health service and local authorities have yet to be fully evaluated.

SPEECH THERAPISTS

Normal communication is a highly complex two-way process which involves a receptive phase (receiving and decoding information) and an expressive phase (the encoding and transmission of information in a comprehensible form). Communication can be verbal, comprising spoken and written language, or non-verbal which includes eye contact, facial expression and gesture. In everyday interactions both types of communication are used simultaneously. When dealing with a person with speech or language impairment it is obviously important to know at what point and to what extent the process has broken down. It is also essential to look at the impairment in terms of the effect it has on the individual, the family and the environment.

Communication impairment

Cerebrovascular disorders (strokes) are the most common cause of specific speech or language problems in the elderly. One third of people who suffer a stroke have speech and/or language problems.

Communication problems can be considered in terms of:

1. disorders of language (dysphasia);
2. disorders of articulation (dyspraxia, dysarthria);

3. disorders of voice (e.g. dysphonia, aphonia) or of fluency (dysfluency).

Dysphasia is the difficulty in encoding and decoding language and hence can be *receptive* (the comprehension of incoming speech is lost and may be gross or subtle) and *expressive* where speech formation is impaired (words may be used repetitively or inappropriately). Receptive and expressive dysphasia often coexist. Dysphasia is usually associated with a *left* hemisphere lesion.

A *dyspraxia* is the difficulty initiating and carrying out voluntary movement (e.g. of the tongue) and hence can affect speech. It results from damage to the parietal lobe.

Dysarthria is the term used to describe impaired articulation,the effects being on the rate and clarity of speech. Causes include stroke, Parkinson's disease, motor neurone disease and multiple sclerosis.

Dysphonia (abnormal voice, e.g. hoarse) can be due to anxiety, vocal abuse, disease (carcinoma of larynx, hypothyroidism) and post surgery. *Aphonia* can be due to neurological conditions or be psychogenic.

Laryngectomy patients are most commonly found in the over-50 age group and can communicate using oesophageal speech or an electronic artificial larnyx.

Dysfluency (stammer) is found in people of all ages. Dysfluency may follow brain trauma.

The speech therapist's role

The role of the speech therapist involves assessment, treatment and management, and advising staff and relatives.

Assessment involves the use of both formal standardized tests and informal procedures. The aim is to investigate:

1. the nature and extent of the communication problem;
2. the remaining intact communication skills;
3. the effects of other factors (e.g. hearing loss, hemianopia, depression);
4. all aspects of the personality and lifestyle of the patient (early contact with relatives and/or friends is therefore essential);
5. other aspects involved (e.g. swallowing) — this may involve detailed investigations and ongoing further assessment, advice and management plans.

Treatment and management, involves retraining and developing speech, language and communication

skills using material which is relevant and of interest to the patient. It also involves introducing alternative means of communication.

Communication charts consist of picture words and letters and may be useful, but they may be too simplistic for some and too complex for others.

Sign systems such as Makaton are taught to some patients. It is most effective for the dysarthric or dysphasic patient with a predominantly expressive problem. A reasonable level of comprehension is needed and mobility in one arm. The people within one's environment must also be taught to use it.

There is a wide range of electronic or battery-powered aids on the market. They come in all shapes and sizes and many are portable. They range from glorified communication charts to computers producing electronic voices (with a strong American accent!). These machines are generally more appropriate for the severely dysarthric client.

Advising staff and relatives about communication. First and most importantly, think in terms of normal everyday communication. If the patient is anxious or tired, receptive and expressive skills are likely to be affected. Ensure you can see and hear each other clearly and try to check that there is a minimum of distraction in terms of noise and activity. Allow plenty of time for information to be absorbed and for the reply. Try not to go from one subject to another too quickly. Beware of talking too slowly or too strangely or it may be you who is creating the communication barrier.

RECOMMENDED FURTHER READING

Bennett G. *Alzheimer's Disease and Other Confusional States.* Macdonald Optima, London, 1989.

Cartwright A, Smith C. *Elderly People, their Medicines and their Doctors.* Routledge, London, 1988.

Durnin JUGA. Nutrition. In: Brocklehurst JC (ed.), *Textbook of Geriatric Medicine and Gerontology,* 3rd edn. Churchill Livingstone, Edinburgh, 1985.

Hooker S. *Caring for Elderly People: Understanding and Practical Help.* Routledge and Kegan Paul, London, 1987.

Isaacs A, Post F (eds). *Studies in Geriatric Psychiatry.* John Wiley, Chichester, 1979.

Mace Rabins, *et al. The 36-Hour Day: Caring at Home for Confused Elderly People.* Age Concern, London, 1988.

Maczka K. *Assessing Physically Disabled people at Home.* Chapman & Hall, London, 1990.

McClymont M, Thomas S, Denham MJ. *Health Visiting and the Elderly.* Churchill Livingstone, Edinburgh, 1986.

Murphy P. *Dementia and Mental Illness in the Old.* Macmillan, London, 1986.

Norton C. *Nursing for Continence.* Beaconsfield Publications, 1986.

O'Malley K (ed.). *Clinical Pharmacology and Drug Treatment in the Elderly.* Churchill Livingstone, Edinburgh, 1984.

Redfern SJ (ed). *Nursing Elderly People.* Churchill Livingstone, Edinburgh, 1986.

Rowlings C. *Social Work with Elderly People.* George Allen and Unwin, 1981.

Smith L. *Physiotherapy with Older People.* Chapman & Hall, London, 1989.

Squires A. *Rehabilitation of the Elderly Patient.* Croom Helm, London, 1990.

Thompson K. *Caring for an Elderly Relative.* Macdonald Optima, London, 1988.

Wagstaff P, Coakley D. *Physiotherapy and the Elderly Patient.* Croom Helm, London, 1988.

Willard and Spackman (eds). *Occupational Therapy,* 7th edn. JP Lippincroft, Philadelphia, 1988.

INDEX

Accident & Emergency, 147, 184
Accidental hypothermia, 108
Acetyl choline, 33
Achlorhydria, 46
Activities of daily living, 29, 75, 78, 79, 158, 201
Acupuncture, 131
Addison's disease, 44, 51
Adult Protective Services, 140
Advocacy, 203
Age pigments, 9
Ageing, 3, 87
  attitudes, 52
  changes, 6
  damage theories, 8
  disease, 3
  extrinsic, 8
  genetic theories, 8
  heterogeneity, 53, 62
  intrinsic, 8
  mechanisms, 8
  politics, 62
  population, 4, 5
  stereotypes, 52, 61
  successful, 53
Ageism, 61
AIDS, 129
Aids and adaptations, 81, 189
Alcohol, 89, 126
  abuse, 47, 93, 126, 138
  withdrawal, 124
Alcoholics Anonymous, 127
Alimentary system, 45
Alkaline phosphatase, 28
Alternating-pressure air mattresses, 105
Aluminium, 94
Alzheimer's disease, 32, 33, 94, 193
  familial, 33
Alzheimer's Disease Society, 95, 193
Amaurosis fugax, 17

Amitriptyline, 123
Amnestic syndromes, 32, 93
Amulree, Lord, 59
Amyloid, 33, 94
Amyloid angiopathy, 94
Anaemia, 13
Analgesics, 95, 131
Andropause, 43
Androstenedione, 42
Angina, 36
Anorexia, 47
Anti-oxidants, 9
Anticholinergic drugs, 100
Anticonvulsant drugs, 28
Antidepressant drugs, 95, 119, 122, 124
Aphakic lenses, 17
Appetite and nutrition in the elderly, 47
Arcus senilis, 15
Arthritis, 138
Aspirin, 152
Assessment scales, 105, 170
Assessments
  institutional care, 65
Astronauts, 27
Atheroma, 35, 36
Atrial fibrillation, 36
Atrophic gastritis, 46
Atrophic vaginitis, 100
Audiogram, 20
Australian lift, 116
Auto-immune disease, 8, 51
Autonomy, 171, 174
Avicenna, 57

Balance, 20, 34
Baroreceptor reflex, 36
Basal ganglia, 31
Bath assistants, 189
Bed blocker, 72
Bed cradle, 106, 115

Behaviour, 32, 52
Behaviour modification, 195
Benign (senile) forgetfulness, 33, 93
Benign polyps, 47
Bereavement, 53, 125, 127
  counselling, 131
Bi-polar illness, 125
Biofeedback techniques, 131
Biological clock, 9
Biphosphonates, 27
Bladder neck obstruction, 99
Bladder tumours, 99
Blood pressure, 6, 35, 36, 81, 178
Bobath technique, 116, 152, 203
Bone, 25
  cortical, 25
  endosteal envelope, 25
  loss, 26
  trabecular, 25
Bowel function, 52
Brain failure, 77
Brain volume, 31
Breath sounds, 40
Breathlessness, 39
British Geriatrics Society, 59
Bruch's membrane, 18
Burns, 114

Calcitonin, 27
Calcium absorption, 27
Campbell de Morgan, 12
Capillary pressure, 104
Carbamazepine, 123
Carcinoma, 51, 178
  basal cell, 11
  breast, 43
  cervix, 178
  colon, 46
  gastric, 46
  lung, 6

prostate, 43
squamous cell, 11
uterine/endometrial, 43
Cardiac output, 35, 36
Cardiovascular system, 35–37
Care plan, 200
Carers, 167, 172–3, 189, 192–3
Cartilage, 29, 38
Case conference, 139, 159
Case finding, 178
Case records, 77
Casualty officer, 138
Cataract, 17
peripheral, 17
Catchment areas, 186
Catecholamines, 119
Catheters, 101, 131, 195
Cellular ageing, 8
Census, 62
Centenarians, 4
Cerebellar disease, 88
Cerebellum, 31
Cerebral haemorrhage, 150
Cerebrovascular accident, 114, 125
Cervical spondylosis, 89
Chaplains, 193
Charter of Rights, 140
Chemotherapy, 131
Chiropody, 82, 168, 177, 193
Chlormethiazole, 92
Chlorpromazine, 125
Choline acetyl transferase, 33
Chondrocytes, 29
Chromosomal abnormalities, 42, 94
Chronological age, 63
Ciliary muscle, 17
Cirrhosis of the liver, 127
Clinical psychologist, 122, 146, 168, 194
Clinker theory, 9
Clock drawing, 151
Clonus, 116
Clouding of consciousness, 78
Cochlea, 19
Cognitive impairment, 78, 146, 194
Cohort, 6
effects, 7, 52
Cohort-sequential studies, 7
Collagen, 8, 11, 25, 26
Collagenase, 29
Colonic diverticulae, 46
Common law, 146
Communication, 21, 158, 163, 201–2
charts, 206
sign systems, 206
Community Care legislation, 64
Community dental service, 196
Community psychiatric nurses, 68, 121, 195
Comprehensive assessment, 75
Comprehensive care, 162
Conductive deafness, 19
Confusion, 33, 91–96, 127, 185
Constipation, 47, 48
Continence, 53
Continence adviser, 99, 168, 195

Contractures, 152
Cortex, 32, 94
atrophy, 33
frontal, 32, 76
functions, 81
occipital, 32
Costal cartilages, 39
Cot-sides, 92
Counselling, 95, 170, 203
Court of Protection, 147
Creutzfeld–Jacob disease, 94
Crisis prevention, 179
Cross-sectional and longitudinal studies, 6
CT brain scan, 94, 151
Cushing's disease, 26, 44
Cutis rhomboidalis nuchae of Jadassohn, 12
Cystocoele, 100

Day care, 204
Day centre, 68, 204
Day hospital, 167–9, 203
psychiatric, 168
Deafness, 124
Death rates, 7
Debridement, 105
Decibels, 20
Dehydration, 24
Delirium, 125
Delirium tremens, 124, 127
Delusions, 93, 124
Demanding behaviour, 194
Dementia, 33, 92, 125, 146
pugilistica, 93
syndromes, 114, 138
Demography, 62
Dental caries, 45
Dentists, 168, 195
Dentition, 49
Dentures, 45, 76
Dependence, 29, 171
Depression, 42, 47, 76, 93, 95, 118–23, 131
causes, 119
DSM-III criteria, 123
management, 121
mechanisms, 119
non-specific management attention to, 121
occurrence, 119
physical illness, 119
recovery, 122–3
risks of death, 119
severity, 121
scales, 121
types, 119
Dermis, 11
Detrusor instability, 99
Developing countries, 5
Diabetes mellitus, 13, 17, 44
neuropathy, 36, 193
Diarrhoea, 101
Diet, 131, 176
Dietitian, 168, 197

Digoxin, 24
Diogenes syndrome, 53, 126
Disabled Living Foundation, 171
Discharge from hospital, 188–91
Discharge summary, 190
Disengagement, 52, 119
District general manager, 199
District nurse, 68, 138, 189
Diuretics, 24, 36
Diversional therapy, 201
Diverticular disease, 46, 47
Dizziness, 20
DNA, 8
Doctors, 197–8
Domestic tasks, 202
Domiciliary care, 204
Dopamine, 33
Doppler studies, 13, 193
Dothiepin, 123
Down's syndrome, 8, 33, 42, 94
Dressing, 80–1
Drop attacks, 88
Drusen, 18
Dubreuilh's elastoma, 12
Duke University longitudinal studies of ageing, 52
Dysarthria, 95, 206
Dysfluency, 206
Dysphagia, 46
Dysphasia, 206
Dysphonia, 206
Dyspraxia, 93, 206
Dysrhythmias, 88

Ear wax, 19
Eastman, 137
Economic prosperity, 62
Ectropion, 15
Education, 7
Elder abuse, 89, 137–40
Electro-convulsive therapy, 119, 122
Elizabeth I, 57
Embryonic development, 31
Emotion, 32
Emotional lability, 95
Enduring power of attorney, 129, 148
Energy use, 8
Entropion, 15
Environment
ward, 76, 122
revolution, 72–3
Epidermis, 11
Epilepsy, 88
Epiphora, 15
Epithelialization, 105
Equipment and adaptations, 171
Ethnicity, 141–4
Euthanasia, 130
Examination, 80
Exercise, 27, 29, 177
Expectation of life, 5

Faecal incontinence, 47, 101
Faecal smearing, 194
Falls, 87–90

causes, 87
occurrence, 87
Familial polyposis coli, 47
Family planning, 5
Feet, 193
Fertility, 5, 62
Fibre, 52
Fibroblasts, 8
Florence Nightingale, 58
Flowtron, 131
Fluoxetine, 123
Fetal posture, 114
Folate deficiency, 48
Folie à deux, 126
Follicle stimulating hormone, 42
Foot care assistant, 193
Footwear, 82
Forgetting, 33
Fractures
    greenstick, 26
Frail elderly schemes, 185
Free radicals, 8, 9

Gait, 34, 81
Gas exchange, 39
Gastric atrophy, 46
Gastric ulcer, 46, 48
Gastrocolic reflex, 46
Gastrostomy, 152
Gene regulation, 9
General (internal) medicine, 164
General dental practitioner, 45
General practitioner, 68, 121, 138, 177,
    189
    new contract, 177
Generalists, 162
Genetics, 94
Geriatric giants, 71, 75
Gerocomice, 57
Gerontoxon, 15
Glial cells, 31
Glaucoma,
    angle-closure, 15
    open angle, 16
Glutathione, 17
Good neighbour, 185
Granulocytes, 50
Grasp reflex, 76
Grey Panthers, 4, 62
Griffiths report, 199
Guardianship, 148
Gut motility, 46

Hachinski score, 95
Haemolytic anaemia, 51
Haemosiderin, 13
Hair, 12
Hallucinations, 93, 119, 124
    hypnogogic, 124
    hypnopompic, 124
Haloperidol, 92, 125
Handedness, 33
Handicap, 4
Hashimoto's thyroiditis, 51
Haversian canals, 25

Hayflick limit, 8
Health centre, 177
Health promotion, 176
Health visitor, 68, 138, 199
Hearing aids, 21, 76, 198
Hearing impairment, 19, 76
Hearing therapists, 198
Henry VIII, 57
Herpes zoster, 51
Hiatus hernia, 46
High technology, 163
Higher cortical function, 81
Hippocampus, 32, 94
Hippocrates, 57, 197
History of geriatric medicine, 57
History taking
    confused patients, 77
HLA, 9
Hoists, 171
Home help, 68, 189
Home visits, 121, 146, 202, 203
Homeostasis, 22–3
Homosexual relationships, 43
Hormone replacement therapy, 27, 43
Hospice, 128–29
Hospital admission
    refusal, 145
    something must be done, 147
Hospital management, 199
Hospital trusts, 200
Housing, 47
    sheltered, 204–5
Housebound people, 28
Howell, Trevor, 59
Human growth hormone, 27
Huntington's disease, 93
Hyaluronic acid, 29
Hypercalcaemia, 27, 28
Hypernatraemia, 24
Hypertension, 36
Hyperthyroidism, 44
Hypocalcaemia, 27
Hypochondriasis, 118
Hypokalaemia, 101
Hypomania, 126
Hyponatraemic, 24
Hypopigmentation, 11
Hypopituitarism, 44
Hypotension, 36
Hypothalamus, 42
Hypothermia, 108–12
Hypothyroidism, 44
Hypoxia, 40, 93

Iatrogenic problems, 24, 179
Immobility, 26, 83–6, 177
Immune system, 50
    cellular, 8, 40, 50
    humoral, 50
Immunization, 176
Impairments
    disabilities and handicaps, 4
Impipramine, 123
Importuning, 118
Incontinence, 77, 97–102, 195

chart, 99
faecal, 101
overflow, 99
pads, 101
stress, 99
urgency, 99
urinary, 195
Indigestion, 52
Individualism, 174
Infant mortality, 5, 62
Infection, 40, 95
Inflammation, 114
Influenza, 176
Informal carers, 63
Informal networks, 67
Institutional care, 53, 64–5, 146, 170,
    173–4, 194–5
Intelligence, 7, 33
Intervertebral discs, 39
Intestinal obstruction, 47
Iris, 16
Iron deficiency, 48
Isolation, 48
Isotretinoin, 13

J wave, 110
Jekyll and Hyde syndrome, 126
Joint contractures, 113–17
Joint flexibility, 28–9
Joint pain, 114

Kendrick battery, 168
Keratoacanthoma, 12
Keratoses, 11
Key workers, 159
Kinsey Report, 52
Korsakoff's syndrome, 93
Kuru, 94
Kyphosis, 39

l-dopa, 36, 124
Labyrinthitis, 20, 89
Lacunar stroke, 150
Language, 93
Large bowel, 46
Left ventricular failure, 36
Leg ulcers, 13
Legal matters, 145–9
Lens, 15
Leonardo da Vinci, 35
Leukoplakia, 45
Libido, 42
Lice, 14
Lichen planus, 14
Life events, 119
Life span, 5
Lifestyle, 176–7
Limbic system, 32
Lip reading, 198
Lipofuscin, 8, 35
Lithium carbonate, 122, 123, 126
Living will, 129–30
Locus coeruleus, 31
Lofepramine, 123
Long-stay beds, 165

Longitudinal studies, 6
Looser's zones, 28
Losses, 53
Luncheon clubs, 204
Lung
　elasticity, 38
　function, 39
　immunology, 39
　structure, 38
　ventilation perfusion, 39
Luteinizing hormone, 42
Lymphocytes, 51
Lymphokines, 51
Lymphomas, 13

Major histocompatability system, 9
Major tranquillizers, 36, 125
Makaton sign system, 206
Malabsorption, 26, 28, 46, 48
Malignant melanoma, 12
Malnutrition, 47, 48, 197
Mammography, 178
Mania, 125–6
Marriage, 6
Mass media, 61
Massage, 131
Meal times, 122, 174
Meals on wheels, 68, 189, 204
Medical day hospitals, 167
Medication, 77, 79
Melancholy, 42
Melanosis coli, 101
Memory, 32, 93
　long-term, 32
　short-term, 32, 76
Memory clinics, 168
Menopause, 42
　male, 43
Menstruation, 42
Mental competence, 146
Mental Health Act (1983), 146
　guardianship, 148
Mental illness, 138
Mental Test Score, 78, 92
Millard, Peter, 59–60
Mini mental state examination, 92
Mitral incompetence, 35
Mobility, 193, 201
Mobility aids, 171–2
Mono-amine oxidase inhibitors, 122
Motivation, 119
Mucosa, 45–6
Multi-infarct dementia, 94–5
Multi-disciplinary assessment, 121
Multi-disciplinary team, 162, 167–168
Multiple pathology, 71, 78, 162, 185
Multiple sclerosis, 94, 114
Muscle strength, 28, 177
Myasthenia gravis, 51
Myocardial infarction, 88, 92
Myoplasty, 106
Myxoedema, 84

Nascher, 58
Nasogastric tube, 152

National Assistance Act (1948), 147, 205
National Health Service & Community
　Care Act 1990, 63
Needs-related, 164
Nerve blocks, 131
Nerve conduction velocity, 34
Neuritic plaques, 94
Neurofibrillary tangles, 33, 94
Neurogenic bladder, 100
Neurogenic bowel, 101
Neurological examination, 81
Neurosurgery, 131
Neurosyphilis, 88
Neurotransmitters, 33, 119
Night sitters, 95
Nominal dysphasia, 78
Nortriptyline, 123
Nucleus basalis of Meynert, 32, 33
Nursing, 168, 189, 200
Nursing homes, 64
Nursing process, 200
Nursing profile, 200
Nutrition, 47–8

Occupational therapy, 81, 122, 168, 189,
　201
Oesophagus, 46
Old Age Psychiatry services, 164–5
Oocytes, 42
Opiates, 124
Orthotics, 114
Osteoarthritis, 29, 84, 88
Osteoblasts, 26
Osteoclasts, 25
Osteomalacia, 27–8, 88, 197
Osteoporosis, 12, 26, 39

Pain, 106, 130–1
Palatal training device, 196
Palliative care, 128–32
　surgery, 131
Parafollicular C cells, 27
Paranoia, 93, 125
　delusions, 119
Paraphrenia, 125
Parathormone, 26, 27
Parathyroid glands, 27
Parietal lobe, 32
Parkinson's disease, 33, 36, 84, 88, 94,
　138, 193
Parkinson's Disease Society, 69, 193
Parotitis, septic, 46
Part 3 homes, 59, 64, 186
Pegasus Airwave mattress, 105
Pemphigus vulgaris, 51
Pencil and paper tests, 81
Penile sheath, 131
Periodontal disease, 45
Peripheral nervous system, 34
Peristaltic contractions, 46
Pernicious anaemia, 46, 88
Person's day, 122, 170–1
Personal hygiene, 201
Pets, 122, 145
Pharmacists, 202

Pharyngeal pouches, 46, 48
Phenelzine, 123
Phobias, 122, 194
Physical capacity, 28
Physiotherapists, 115, 168, 189, 202–3
Pick's disease, 93
Pilocarpine, 16
Pituitary–adrenal axis, 44
Pleural calcification, 40
Pneumonia, 91, 176
Poor Laws, 58, 71
Population projections, 62
Positron emission tomography, 119
Post-micturition dribble, 100
Postmenopausal osteoporosis, 43
Postural hypotension, 37, 88
Posture, 34
Poverty, 47, 112
Power of Attorney, 148
Pre-pemphigoid, 14
Presbycusis, 19
Presbyoesophagus, 46
Presbyopia, 16–17
Presentation of disease, 70–73
Pressure sores, 103–7, 115, 152
Prevention, 105, 176
Primary health care, 163
Privacy, 76
Private care, 165, 205
Problem list, 75
Problem orientated medical records, 197
Progeria, 8
Programmed ageing, 9
Prostatism, 43, 100
Proteoglycans, 29
Proximal myopathy, 28, 88
Pruritus, 12–13
Pseudobulbar palsy, 95
Pseudelirium, 92
Pseudodementia, 93, 121
Psychiatric hospitals, 121
Psychiatrists, 168
Psychomotor skills, 122
Psychosis, 92
Psychotherapy, 122
Ptosis, 15
Pulmonary emboli, 95
Purchaser/provider separation, 199
Pythagoras, 57

Quality of life, 130

Radiotherapy, 131
Reality orientation, 100, 195
Records, 158
Rectum, 49, 99
　bleeding, 47, 138
　examination, 47, 81
Rectangularization of survival, 5–6
Referral, 160, 186
Rehabilitation, 4, 29, 159–160, 167, 170
Relaxation, 131, 177
Renal dialysis, 163
Renal tubule, 28
Residential homes, 205

Respiration
    abdominal, 40
    airways, 38
    alveoli, 38
    diaphragm, 38
    muscles, 39
    rate, 40, 81
    airways resistance, 28
Respite care, 173, 193
Retention of urine, 47
Retinal artery occlusion, 17
Retinal detachment, 17
Retinal vein occlusion, 17
Rewarming, 111
Rewarming collapse, 111
Rheumatoid arthritis, 12, 51
Risk of death, 7
Rocking chair syndrome, 52

Saliva, 45
Salivary glands, 45
Sacks, Oliver, 32
Saunders, Cicely, 128–9
Schizophrenia, 125, 126
Screening, 139, 177–8
Scurvy, 26, 48, 197
Section 47 (of National Assistance Act),
    147
Selenium, 9
Senile macular degeneration, 17
Senile plaques, 94
Senile purpura, 12
Senile pruritus, 12
Serotonin (5-HT), 119, 122
Services
    age-related, 60, 164
    geriatric styles, 164
    informal carers, independent sector, 63
    local authority, health authority, 64
    social security, housing departments,
      64
Severe weather payments, 112
Sex, 52, 77
Sheltered housing, 204–5
Shy–Drager syndrome, 36
Skeleton, 25
Small bowel, 46
Smoking, 6, 39, 47, 127, 176
Snellen chart, 76
Social admissions, 71
Social contacts, 119
Social emergencies, 186
Social engagement, 53
Social networks, 67, 72, 179, 185
Social presentation of disease, 71
Social reports, 204
Social work, 122, 168
Social worker, 68, 189, 203
Socio-economic development, 5, 62
Somatic mutation, 9
Space blanket, 111

Spasticity, 114, 115
Speech, 19, 33
Speech therapists, 152, 168, 205
Spider naevi, 12
Splinter haemorrhage, 12
Spurious diarrhoea, 47
Stair lifts, 172
Steatorrhoea, 46
Steroids, 124
Stomach, 46
Stones, 99
Stress, 177
Stroke, 93, 95, 124, 126, 138, 150–4, 178
    acute management, 151
    communication, 205–6
    complications, 152
    diagnosis, 150
    follow-up, 152
    prognosis, 153
    recovery, 152
    recurrence, 152
    rehabilitation, 152
    severity, 152
    speech, 152
    swallowing, 152
Successful ageing, 53
Suicide, 119
Support systems, 178
Surveillance, 178
Survival, 5, 7, 39
Synovial joints, 113
Syphilis, 94

Tabes dorsalis, 88
Tardive dyskinesia, 126
Teamwork, 4, 157–8
    primary health care, 160
Teeth, 45, 81
Telangiectasia, 12
Temperature
    core, 108
    oral, 51
    rectal, 112
    regulation, 109
Temporal lobe, 32
Terminal care, 128
Tetanus, 176
Thalamus, 32
Therapeutic milieu, 194
Thermoregulation, 36
Thiamine, 127
Thirst, 24
Thioridazine, 92
Thymus gland, 9, 51
Thyroid gland, 44
Thyrotoxicosis, 44
Tintern Abbey, 57
Tissue grafts, 51
Tobacco, 127
Toilet management, 201
Traditional remedies, 79

Training, 39, 163
Transcutaneous nerve stimulation, 131
Transient global amnesia, 93
Transparent skin syndrome, 12
Transport, 177
Tricyclic antidepressants, 122
Trisomy chromosome, 42
Tuberculosis, 40, 51
Tunnel vision, 16

Ulcerative colitis, 47
Ultra-violet (U/V) light, 11–12, 28
Unit general manager, 199
Unrecognized disease, 178
Uraemia, 14
Urinary incontinence, see Incontinence
Urinary tract infection, 91, 100
Urine, 99
Urodynamic clinic, 100
Uterine prolapse, 100
Uterus, 43

Vacuoles, 33
Vagina, 43, 138
    examination, 81, 99
Vasovagal attacks, 88
Venous stasis, 13
Vertigo, 20, 88
Vibration sense, 34
Visual acuity, 81
Visual impairments, 76, 124, 177
Vitamin B_{12}, 48, 88
Vitamin C, 8, 48, 106
Vitamin D, 27
Vitreous opacities (floaters), 17

Walking, 81
Walking frames, 172
Walking stick, 82, 172
Wandering, 194
Warren, Marjorie, 58
Wernecke–Korsakoff's syndrome, 127
Wheelchairs, 82, 171
Wills, 145
Women, 5–6, 53
Workhouse life, 58
World Wars, 6, 63
Wrinkling, 11
WRVS (Womens Royal Voluntary
    Service), 204

X-ray
    chest, 38, 40
    osteoporosis, 26

Young old, 63
Young people, 61
Youth culture, 61

Zinc, 106